# THE
# HOMEMADE
# MD

A PRACTICAL, DO-IT-YOURSELF APPROACH
TO NAVIGATING TODAY'S HEALTHCARE SYSTEM.

## ARDEN BALLARD
### MS, PA-C, ATC

For more information, email thehomemademd@gmail.com
ISBN:
Paperback: 979-8-9899597-0-9
Hardback: 979-8-9899597-1-6

To get the best experience when utilizing a book of this type, I've found readers who download and use the FREE Resource guide are able to implement faster and take the next steps necessary to become one's own Homemade MD. If that's not incentive enough, get a free gift when you order a copy of this useful and informative book.

You can get a copy by visiting:
**www.thehomemademd.com**

This book is dedicated to those I couldn't help, to those to whom I didn't provide my best effort, and to those I simply disappointed. I write this as an imperfect provider, and while I see patients to the best of my ability, I know there were days where I simply didn't have my best to give. You came to me in a time of need, and I couldn't meet you in your space.

My prayer is that the words in this book can help at least one person overcome, at a minimum, even one obstacle in the often intimidating and confusing healthcare industry. If I achieved that goal, then this book, to me, is an overwhelming success.

# TABLE OF CONTENTS

# INTRODUCTION

## WHY DO WE NEED A

## HOMEMADE MD?

Do you remember your first computer? I was about 10 years old. I was given a "new" surplus computer from one of my mother's friends. I was so excited to unbox this monstrosity, this behemoth of silicone and steel. I was kind of an aspiring nerd, and I'd eventually ruin the heck out of this computer by installing games and deleting super important files to make room for these useless applications.

This thing was HUGE. It took up the entire desk, and it had to weigh 30 pounds. And the monitor...oh the monitor! The old tube design was easily deeper than the desk itself. Using the term "color" was a stretch, as the reds, greens, and blues would flicker and sputter to life. It wasn't pretty, but at least it was mine. And I learned a lot from navigating this primitive personal computing device.

You're probably asking, "What the heck does this have to do with medicine?" In my opinion, everything. It's a metaphor for the big rat's nest of a system that we have created.

Today's American healthcare system is immense. It's a monster that is rapidly growing out of control. The 2020 Global Consumer Healthcare Market size was valued at $3.3 trillion in 2020 and is projected to reach $6.6 trillion by 2028. $3.3 and $6.6 *trillion*.

A big machine isn't necessarily a bad thing. Like the computer of my youth, the size wasn't the issue. The complexity of the machine, coupled with the fact that the man (or boy) in the driver's seat had no idea what he was doing with it, made for a complete mess.

There are many well-intended providers and caregivers in the medical community, but where there is a share of $3.3 trillion on the table, there are corporations and political entities aiming to take all they can for personal and corporate gain. The larger the system, the larger the complexity and, in my experience, the greedier.

My point is the system doesn't care about you, the individual patient. That's right; They. Don't. Care. Yes, you probably know of the privately owned primary care practice, or urgent care facilities, that takes the time to sit down with their patients, gets to know them, treats them right. But today's healthcare model seeks those clinics and buys them. They want them for the client list. They come in and offer good money, promise to "take care of the staff," implement their Electronic Health Record (EHR) and computer software, and they slap their name and branding on the building. Sometimes, the provider stays, and sometimes they retire. They may relocate and open another clinic. The ultimate result is yet another private entity is devoured by the "big guy."

What does this mean for the provider? These providers become giant walking stress balls. They become overworked, overburdened, overstressed. They are underappreciated and underpaid. Referring back the computer analogy, it's as if you kept that sucker on for three months, grinding and computing and stressing it to its limits. Dust gathers and clogs its fans, generating heat and becoming increasingly more inefficient over time. "The job must be done," the computer would say if it could talk. This was, after all, 1994, and the computer would start to audibly whine and strain, until eventually, it would cease to perform.

Providers today go nonstop. There are Relative Value Units (RVUs), a convoluted system to describe provider reimbursement, to be earned, charts to complete on that fancy new computer and EHR that most providers — especially the experienced ones — can't understand or refuse to learn. There are patient phone calls to make, insurance authorizations to complete, and discussions to have with the plethora of administrators that entice the practitioner to the "dark" side. These folks typically have zero experience with practicing medicine. A college business degree, or a "Healthcare MBA," gives them the "authority" to oversee providers who spent decades learning the art and science of patient care. The administrators that do have experience in patient care are usually disconnected from the present-day life of a full-time provider. Not always, but most provider/administrator types chose that path to escape the daily grind of full-time patient care.

That computer I received sure did make things convenient, but that convenience included a hefty price tag. The computer isn't able to think in shades of gray, only black and white, zeros and ones. The problem with that is medicine was built on the backs of providers who *lived* thinking in the gray. Asking "what if." Challenging the "way things were always done."

I'm just scratching the surface of my 15-plus years of medical experience, but if I can define it in just one phrase, it would be one that a good friend of mine Greg Anderson once told me:

### "No One is Coming to Save You"

As the system gets bigger, more complex, less personal, and the population continues to expand, grow more unhealthy and more dependent on others, the information that follows becomes extremely important. Critical, in fact. The American average wait time for

Emergency Medical Services (EMS) to arrive at a scene is about 15 minutes. Not only can that seem like 18 lifetimes to those involved in the crisis, it could also mean the death of the one waiting on the service. What if you had an inkling, a sliver of knowledge about the situation? What if you could aid in the prevention of said emergency, or notice the symptoms before they became so critical?

That, my new friend, is the purpose of this book.

It's time someone offered you some knowledge. I want to help you navigate the rough seas of today's complex healthcare system. Consider this book a fresh sail, some great paddles, and providing a little self-confidence. If I can prevent one phone call into the system, prevent one unnecessary trip to the hospital or urgent care (I'm talking to you, Mr. "I go to the ER [Emergency Room] with my cold." We'll discuss you soon.), save you a few bucks in your pharmacy, or save you precious time when it comes to a life or death situation, then this book, to me, is akin to a medical manual. That said, let's be clear; I'm not *your* provider, I'm not diagnosing *your* specific medical problem, and I'm not telling you what to do or how to act. Don't sue me, I'm just your friendly neighborhood good Samaritan. I don't replace quality medical care; we will cover what that actually looks like.

You're probably wondering, "Who is this bozo crapping on the healthcare industry?" Hi. I'm Arden Ballard, physician assistant, certified athletic trainer, and victim of the healthcare burnout phenomenon. I started my career as an athletic trainer in 2007 and continued my education to become a physician assistant. Since 2010, I've been treating patients in a large variety of settings. I've consulted patients in ERs and urgent care clinics. I've worked alongside surgeons in operating rooms, and I've seen tens of thousands of patients in an outpatient clinic setting. I've had tough, life-changing conversations with patients. I've taught at conferences and lectured in classrooms. I've seen firsthand what "the system" can do to a provider, and I've personally fallen victim to burnout.

All I ever wanted to do is help people. Considering how healthcare is currently practiced, I believe this book is the best way to do it.

This book should result in more money in your pocket, more time on your watch, and a more pleasant experience while you're navigating the healthcare system. Not only will I discuss common medical diagnoses and touch on the most common visit types, I'll also give you some insight on how to navigate your healthcare network, understand your insurance and how it works behind the scenes, and how to stock your medicine cabinet at home. Preparation is key, and an ounce of prevention is still worth a pound of cure and in some cases, tons.

While this book is not, by any means, a substitute for medical care, the knowledge in this book should empower you to make wise decisions for you and your loved ones when it comes to your medical decision making. It'll save you time, money, and headaches.

This is my guarantee to you: I promise that reading this book will teach you something. Something that has the potential to save a life. If this book doesn't offer you any value whatsoever, burn it. Send me the ashes. I'm happy to take the heat. (Spoiler Alert: You're going to learn something.)

This information isn't taught in schools. Most of this book consists of discussions I've had with my patients at one point in my career. Even if you took a health class in high school, can you recall a single topic you discussed? I went to a great high school, and we didn't have a class dedicated to practical, applied medical knowledge. I want you to have practical medical understanding oozing from your ears at the end of this book. And if you love it, tell me. If you hate it, tell me that also. It's time to dive in and see how you may be empowered to save someone's life. That's right; even you, Ms. "I'm scared of blood" and Mr. "I don't know my stomach from my left foot," I got you covered. Let's begin.

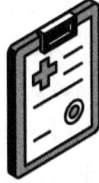

# CHAPTER 1

## CRITICAL THINKING CAN SAVE YOUR LIFE

*Have more humility. Remember you don't know the limits of your own abilities. Successful or not, if you keep pushing beyond yourself, you will enrich your own life, and maybe even please a few strangers.*

–A.L. Kennedy

My athletic training program didn't begin until my junior year in college. It was a five-semester program geared toward training "certified athletic trainers," i.e., medical professionals that specialize in the prevention, assessment, and rehabilitation of athletic injuries. My school had a terrific program at the time, and I was excited and eager to begin.

I was also a bit hubristic and proud of my accomplishments thus far in my collegiate career. I was a top notch student and heavily involved on campus, and I thought I knew it all; what 21-year-old male doesn't?

On the first day of my athletic training program, I learned my first lesson of medicine, and an important life lesson in general—humility. As our class walked from the classroom building to the athletic complex, we noticed a student laying on the ground, face down, screaming in pain. Some of us sprang into action, assessing the troubled college student and attempting to collect details of his issue. We were able to reduce his terror from a scream to a panicked conversation, and that's when we heard the fear in his voice: "I fell from the balcony, and I can't feel my arms or legs."

We didn't know what to do. Sure, we were educated on the anatomy of the body and had some (albeit very little) practical knowledge on how to apply it, but none of us had been in this situation before. It felt as if we all stood there for an eternity, staring at each other. It was then that our professor casually walked out of the athletic building and waved to us. "Hi class," the professor said, calm and collected, "What are y'all up to?"

We were all hovered around this boy on the concrete, speechless. He must have seen the concern on our faces, and he replied, "So what are you going to do about our friend here?"

That's when most of us realized today's lesson; our professor brought us here to perform. He set up the whole performance to mimic a real scenario.

Our "patient" was a graduate assistant from upstairs. He didn't fall. Rather, the professor selected him to be our live test subject. He stood at a distance, assessing our thought process, keeping us calm, and when we would get stuck, he'd ask a question to encourage our thinking and teamwork skills. "You got the board; what should you do with it? How should you move forward? What is the safest move for your patient?" He couldn't help himself and added some pressure, occasionally yelling, "Hurry up!" or, "You're taking way too long!"

We spent the majority of the 90-minute class fumbling through the Emergency Action Plan (EAP), i.e., calling 911, collecting the spine board from the building, rolling the patient, applying the spine board, and securing the patient for emergency transport. When the patient was secured to the board, the professor stepped in to conclude the exercise, and our previously paralyzed patient unstrapped himself from the board and stood next to the professor. We were mentally and physically exhausted.

"That took you guys just over an hour. It took 15 students one hour to backboard one person." We stood quietly in the brisk air, understanding the severity of the issue we just experienced. We all thought we were big shots for getting accepted into the program, and with one class and one patient, we were brought to our knees with the realization that we had a lot to learn.

Personally, that day was less about the medical knowledge we learned and more about the critical thinking skills that were planted, and later developed skills that help me through every shift I work and every patient I see. Critical thinking is a vital skill for any healthcare professional, regardless of their specialty. It allows you to make sound decisions, solve problems, and communicate effectively with patients. I am still humbled on a daily basis at work, taking a deep breath and organizing the tasks in order keep *me* calm, and that makes for a calm patient. I do not write this book to equip you with the vast range of medical knowledge. I wrote it so that you will be prepared when your child falls off their bike and breaks their arm, or when your mother is diagnosed with a debilitating (or terminal) illness. How will you react? What will be your response? Let's discuss a few mindset tips to keep you on track and positive so you're ready when it counts.

It'd be easy for me to begin by saying, "Stay calm in stressful situations," but you didn't buy my book for that. While staying calm is a fundamental pillar in all forms of healthcare, let me elaborate. I have a personal "10 second rule" when it comes to reacting to trauma, like a kid falling off a bike, for example. If I witness an accident or injury, 10 seconds is a long time for the person to react in a way that will give me a good idea about that person's status. At 10 seconds, a child may have brushed themselves off and resumed play, or they could be holding their knee and crying. The soccer player that just had a head-on collision with another player could still be unconscious, or they could have jumped up and gotten back in the game. The reaction that will get you in trouble is the immediate, knee-jerk, spring- to-action response. Don't rush to the field of play or give the patient an anxiety attack by signaling to them, "Holy cow, you should be hurt right now." The 10 second rule has saved me from a lot of embarrassing moments. Remember: If it's broken right now, it'll be broken 10 seconds from now.

This next one is a little tougher, especially if it's your friend or sibling. In the moment, try to remove yourself from any personal connection you may have. If this person is truly injured, or if the matter is one of life or death, your feelings about the person will only lead to anxiety and indecision. While this might sound difficult or nearly impossible to achieve, it starts with that first deep breath and those first 10 seconds. While I'm counting to 10 in my brain, I'm reminding myself to keep calm. I'm also flipping through my knowledge base and thinking about how I need to prepare myself. Did the person land awkwardly on their leg? Perhaps I should grab supplies for a makeshift splint or crutches. Did they land on their head? I should proceed with caution if they remain on the ground, careful not to inadvertently move them and cause further damage. The one thing I am *not* thinking about is, "Oh, my poor little boy! What am I going to do?" When seconds and minutes matter, there is no room for drama.

I'll add one more important trait to consider when it comes to a proper mindset when dealing with patients: Empathy. No matter the age or disposition of the patient, if you can put yourself in their shoes for a second and feel what they're feeling, you'll handle the situation far greater than if you were to just think about yourself in the situation. The best providers know what the patient is feeling before the patient knows what they're feeling.

Logical thinking is critical to a successful outcome. Embarrassingly, I have had my moments where I throw logic out the window and act out of emotion. When my second son was soon to be born, there was a hurricane approaching southeast Louisiana where we live. Concerned for the well-being of my wife and child, I remember calling my wife while we were both at work. "Honey, if the storm hits, and we can't get to your doctor's hospital (about a 30-minute drive for us), what are we going to do? Where are we going to go?" My wife, being the calm and logical bride that she is, simply said, "Arden, we'll go to the nearest hospital. There just happens to be one essentially in our backyard," she said with a chuckle. I could feel her eyes rolling through the phone. And of course, like usual, she was right; we could essentially walk there. We actually delivered our first child there, but due to a change in insurance, we had to change hospitals.

But the answer she gave wasn't sufficient for me. I blame "Dad Brain." It's a thing; you can Google it. Completely dissatisfied with her answer, I told her that I didn't appreciate her tone, and I'll call the OBGYN floor at the hospital to get their opinion. "Go right ahead," she said, actively laughing at this point. "Fine!" I said, as I hung up the phone and dialed the hospital.

"I need to speak to the Labor and Delivery charge nurse please," I said as the operator picked up. If any of you know a charge nurse, I'll give you an insight into their personality; they don't put up with nonsense. Most of the time, their conversations are short and to the point. They have enough going on, and if you ask a dumb question, they'll let you'll know. Some of the nicest nurses I've ever worked with are charge nurses, but they'll let you have it.

And this one let me have it.

"L&D this is Jane," she said, seemingly all in one syllable.

"Hey, this is Arden. My wife is supposed to come in this week, but I'm worried about this storm. What's the best protocol if we can't get there?"

There was a pause, then a sigh. "Arden, if you can't get to *our* hospital to deliver your child, you then go to the nearest hospital." The way she said it made the entire situation crystal clear, and I realized how absolutely crazy I must sound.

"Um, sure. Of course. Thanks Jane," I said, tail between my legs. I didn't call my wife back right away, but she certainly used the opportunity to call *me*. She got a great laugh out of it, and I still can't live this story down.

I tell this tale to remind you that we're all human and we sometimes let thoughts, events, and emotions cloud our better judgment. Especially in times of stress and heightened emotions, we don't think clearly. As previously mentioned, it's important to take a step back and observe the situation objectively. Had I been Jane and received that phone call from a stranger, I would have probably given them a similar explanation. Emergencies require emergent care, and that would be at the nearest location you can get to.

What are some of those emergencies, you ask? Let's address some of the obvious ones here:

- Does your patient look lifeless? No pulse or reaction?
- Does your patient (you or a loved one) have facial drooping, slurred speech, or can't move an arm or a leg?
- Do they have a problem with their airway, i.e. they can't breathe?
- Do they have a bone/limb pointing in the wrong direction?
- Did they develop sudden, squeezing chest pain, shortness of breath, excessive sweating, pale?

These issues deserve attention. In the following chapters, we will address how to handle these situations from a generalized approach. I don't expect you to be able to pick up a stethoscope and save the day, per se, but having a clear head, a logical, systematic approach, and acting swiftly and safely may just save this person's life.

Humility is an important trait in these situations as well. It's completely okay to not know what to do. No one in the medical community expects you to know what took us years of study and experience to grasp. Doing only what's in our control and capability is far safer than trying to be the hero and doing something inappropriately. As we dive into the core of this book, I want you to approach the content with a sense of calmness and humility. It's really easy to get upset in these circumstances. The right mindset will help you navigate the medical community with ease. With the right mindset, you will be amazed at what you can handle.

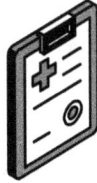

# CHAPTER 2
## THE HOSPITAL SYSTEM

*America's healthcare system is neither healthy, caring, nor a system.*

–Walter Cronkite

I will never forget the first patient I ever evaluated as a physician assistant student. I was assigned to an inpatient psychiatry unit in Trenton, New Jersey . Having never stepped foot in New Jersey, my roommate and best friend drove us to our first day as "clinical year" students. We were really excited, but there was some obvious tension and nervousness among us as we hit the road in his old Honda Accord.

As we got settled and completed our orientation, the coordinator walked us to our unit and got straight to work. My friend was assigned to the ER for the day. They had an ER strictly for psychologically ill patients. I was assigned to the inpatient unit where people spend days to weeks undergoing a rigorous rehabilitation process.

There was one thing I noticed the second I put my belongings down; this place was *locked down*. There were plenty of security guards (plural)–at least three I saw offhand–and shatter-proof glass surrounding the nurses' station where we would do our charting. The patients would walk around the station and peer inside. Some would ask for food, some would strike up a conversation. But within minutes of me sitting down, I noticed several agitated and angry patients. One thing was apparent: These patients didn't want to be there.

I was handed my first patient chart. I'm old enough to say that I came from a "paper chart" era, before EHRs were commonplace, and I was astonished when I was handed this mountain of a paper chart. It was a maroon colored three-ring binder that was about five inches thick. The corners were frayed, and there were color tabs protruding from the sides and top of the binder. I was definitely nervous

I was asked to get a feel for who the patient was and perform an initial evaluation. I read over the chart for what seemed like days. I learned that this patient is no stranger to the unit, having been admitted dozens of times over the past few years. The patient recently admitted he believed that he was Michael Jackson. He has returned from the dead with one goal in mind; to kill his family.

I was sweating, trembling, and *not* comfortable with my assignment. "At least I know I am not cut out to work in psychiatry," I thought to myself. After collecting my thoughts and wiping my brow, I walked around the corner and into the exam room to interview this patient.

"Hello, my name is Arden. I'm one of the physician assistant students here to talk to you." I managed to form a complete sentence, which I perceived as a victory. "How's your day going?" I peered over the chart and across the room into this man's eyes. He was mythical in size. He made John Coffey (the inmate from *The Green Mile*)[1] look like a hamster by comparison. He was a gigantic human, with muscle mass that would rival a professional bodybuilder. He had a shaved head and was likely 6 feet 5 inches tall. He looked tall even as he sat in the chair across from me. Despite his size, he continued to insist that he was Michael Jackson. He even grabbed a white latex glove from the wall and wore it on his right hand.

"I'm here, aren't I?" He replied, clearly not interested in entertaining my questions. "What are we here for today?" I really had no idea how to start this conversation; remember, I was *very* new to this type of thing.

He paused and looked down at his hand. He didn't say anything for a few seconds, something that certainly increased my already elevated anxiety. As soon as I began opening my mouth to ask something else, he looked up and replied, "Is that my chart in your hand?". "Um, yes. Yes it is." His eyes got wide and he grit his teeth. "Then you know why I'm here. It's in my fucking chart."

I promptly excused myself from the room.

I experienced so many emotions that day, including thoughts along the lines of, "What did I get myself into?" I considered not going back, but after discussion with my buddy on the way home, I mustered the confidence to return the following day. To my surprise, the patient was gone. I asked our supervising doctor where he went, and was told that he met the criteria to follow up with his outpatient psychiatrist. They let him go!

This was my first insight to "the system" of healthcare. This patient was clearly sick and in need of help. Was he offered the help he needed and refused it? Was the system simply giving up on him? The answer is probably somewhere in the middle, but the fact remains that the system has some major flaws.

The English language defines "system" as (1) a set of things working together as parts of a mechanism or an interconnecting network, (2) a set of principles or procedures according to which something is done, i.e., an organized framework or method. When I refer to a "hospital system," I'm mainly referring to a network of buildings, providers, clinics, hospitals, etc., with the same name slapped on the side of it. They typically use the same EMR and computer programs, have some sort of board of directors or executive administrators that control the inner and outer workings of the brand and work under a set of guidelines laid out by the aforementioned administrators.

In the U.S., most people believe these hospital systems are the premier medical facilities in the country. We don't have many "old school" private practice physicians left. In today's healthcare world, it's hard to run a competitive private medical practice yourself. Margins are far slimmer than people imagine. When margins are slim, there is increased pressure to see more patients. When over 30% of the medical doctors in the U.S. are over 60[2], there's less interest to take on more patients and work harder for the same, or less, revenue.

This brings up a point that I'll mention now: Medicine is a business. There are caring people in healthcare, but the hospital is a business. Make no mistake about it.

People forget this all the time, but the systems haven't. The systems often keep a watchful eye on these older private practices. They aren't studying their competition. They're strategically positioning themselves to buy them out, specifically to buy their patient log. Hospital systems want your information, and they want your doctor. They will offer these practices top dollar (and then some) to sell their practice in order to reach their patients. They will give them a cash out option, give them a plush job for a few years, and they will tell them, "You won't have to work as hard. You can enjoy the twilight of your career and retire off into the sunset."

Does it always end so glamorously for the practice owner? I presume the results will vary. But what I can tell you is that, in my personal opinion, these systems aren't in the business primarily to serve their patients and their community. They're in it to *make money*. Did you know that there are about 16 healthcare workers for every doctor in the U.S.? Ten of those 16 are administrators.[3] That means there are 16 people that rely on every doctor to pay their salaries.

This creates a business model that relies heavily on patient volume. In other words, get 'em in, get 'em out. Add the ever-increasing complexities such as billing and coding requirements, insurance reimbursement and political changes, laws and rules, you have a machine that needs myriad attention. That patient log we talked about? Ms. Judy is no longer Ms. Judy; she's medical record number N1242863. When she goes to see her usual primary care doctor, she's shocked to see she's been reassigned to the stable of providers in the same specialty. The provider she sees is part of this well-oiled machine and has their exam down to a prompt four minutes. There is zero personalization. The system takes humanity out of medicine, whether they mean to or not. This system is a big pond, and you're only one small fish.

Again, I don't insinuate that all providers and healthcare professionals are sterile, careless machines that have ice water flowing through their veins. However, the state of the healthcare system as a whole does not typically warrant sufficient time to develop relationships with their patients. This is one of my personal gripes as a provider. I got into medicine to help people, to make a difference. I had these ideas of touching lives and making an impact, after observing most patients leave their respective provider's offices confused and frustrated. Their trust in the system has been shaken. They pay twice as much than any other patient with lackluster results. Most providers leave the office drained and without the personal satisfaction they believed they would receive. They are stressed beyond belief.

What does all this have to do with you? It's more important than ever to have a working knowledge of the system and be your own healthcare advocate as well as for your loved ones.

The first thing I want you to consider is carrying a backup of your medical records. As amazing as today's electronic medical record (EMR) systems are, there is one fatal flaw: The programs do not talk to each other, therefore, there is a huge gap in communications between potential providers and staff. If you go to hospital A, and they use one EMR, then you go to hospital B six months later (with a different EMR), and the latter has no idea what happened during that former visit.

Just like you shouldn't drive across the country without a spare tire, you shouldn't traverse healthcare systems without a backup of your records. My first gift to you is a template of this document. This document can be downloaded and printed, stored on a computer or your phone, or you can keep it on the drive and access it on any device in real time. This document is intended to offer a "snapshot" of your medical history for anyone that needs to see it. This includes your current insurance information, your chronic medical conditions, all medications you take, including prescription and over-the-counter (OTC) medicines and supplements, allergies (food and otherwise), past surgeries and procedures, your drinking, smoking and/or drug history and important resources. To get this document, go to www. thehomemademd.com/EAP.

## 1. Personal Information

| Full Name | Date of Birth | Gender |
|---|---|---|
| | | |

| Address | Emergency Contact(s) | Primary Phone Number |
|---|---|---|
| | • Name: _____<br>• Relationship: _____<br>• Phone Number: _____ | |

## 2. Medical History

| Chronic Conditions (e.g., diabetes, hypertension) | Allergies: (medications, food, others) | Blood Type (if known) |
|---|---|---|
| | | |

## 3. Previous Surgical History

| List of Surgeries: (Include name/type of surgery and approximate dates) |
|---|
| |

## 4. Current Medications

| Name of Medication | Dosage | Frequency | Purpose (e.g., blood pressure, diabetes) |
|---|---|---|---|
| | | | |

## 5. Physician(s) and Healthcare Providers

| Primary Care Physician | Specialists: Type (e.g., Cardiologist), |
|---|---|
| • Name: _____<br>• Contact Information: _____ | • Name: _____<br>• Contact Information: _____ |

## 6. Local Hospitals and Medical Facilities

| Preferred Hospital | Alternate Hospital | Pharmacy |
|---|---|---|
| • Name: _____ | • Name: _____ | • Name: _____ |
| • Relationship: _____ | • Relationship: _____ | • Relationship: _____ |
| • Phone Number: _____ | • Phone Number: _____ | • Phone Number: _____ |

## 7. Health Insurance Information

| Provider Name | Policy Number | Group Number (if applicable) | Contact Number for Verification |
|---|---|---|---|
| _____ | _____ | _____ | _____ |

## 8. Advanced Directives

| Resuscitation Preferences (CPR/DNR) | Living Will (brief summary and where to find the full document) | Healthcare Power of Attorney (contact information if different from emergency contact) |
|---|---|---|
| _____ _____ | _____ _____ _____ _____ | _____ |

## 9. Miscellaneous Information

| Language Preference | Special Instructions (e.g., pacemaker, hearing aids, disabilities | Religious Considerations (if relevant to medical care) |
|---|---|---|
| _____ | _____ _____ _____ | _____ _____ _____ |

### 10. Consent Statement for Emergency Use

I,................................................. hereby authorize any emergency medical personnel, first responders, or healthcare providers to use the information provided in this document for the purposes of medical treatment and emergency care. This document is intended to communicate my medical history, current medications, healthcare preferences, and contact information for my primary care and emergency contacts in situations where I am unable to communicate for myself. I understand that this document contains sensitive personal health information and it is my responsibility to ensure its accuracy and safekeeping. I agree to update this information regularly to reflect any changes in my medical condition, treatment preferences, or emergency contacts.
This consent is given voluntarily and without coercion. I understand that I have the right to revoke this consent at any time, except to the extent that action has been taken in reliance on it.

Signature: _____

Date: _____

This template will come in handy if you are ever admitted to the hospital for an illness or procedure. Once you're in the hands of the hospital, your current "medication list" will inevitably be a little unreliable. It will be important to update it once you are discharged and when you follow up with your primary care provider (PCP).

This document needs to be "alive," meaning it needs to be kept up-to-date and accurate. Share it with your loved one or person responsible for your health. Not only will your provider have a huge smile on their face once they see it, it will save you time, and it could potentially save your life.

Next, I want you to use the hospital system's resources to your advantage. You're paying for it, you may as well use it. If you are in their hospital as a patient, they likely have case managers, social workers, nutritionists, and more at your disposal. While some of these services may have fees associated with them, these groups offer loads of free services for you to take advantage of. Allow me to introduce you to some of them here.

Case management, as defined by the Case Management Society of America (CMSA)[4], "is a collaborative process of assessment, planning, facilitation, care coordination, evaluation, and advocacy for options and services to meet an individual's and family's comprehensive health needs through communication and available resources to promote patient safety, quality of care, and cost-effective outcomes."

You're probably asking yourself, "What the heck does that mean?" I know I did, and I've worked in medicine for 15 years.

The bottom line is case managers help you juggle all the complex hospital red tape and coordinate your plan of care with you, your family, and the doctor(s) and hospital(s) that are involved. In the hospital, their role might include assessing your health insurance and coordinating the best—and least expensive—plan of action with the doctors and hospitals. Health insurance companies also hire case managers[5], and they work to ensure you're getting quality, medically necessary healthcare fast and at a reasonable cost. If you're in the hospital, and you haven't been offered to speak to a case manager, speak up. Either ask your nurse, or you or a loved one, to call your insurance company. Nowadays, I'm all about having a team of people in your corner. If the hospital can have lawyers and administrators trying to get as much out of the patient, then the patient needs people that can speak intelligently on their behalf and defend them.

A medical social worker[6] is also a valuable resource during your hospital experience. Communication between providers and patients is never adequate. When the average visit concludes in minutes, there is no doubt questions that aren't asked, or aren't even considered, by the time the provider is out the door. The social worker's role in the hospital revolves primarily around discharge planning and aiding in the family's preparation for life after the hospital stay. This could include answering other questions regarding the particular diagnosis and what to expect when you leave the hospital.

More important than understanding all these ancillary services is understanding what you should do with them. First, if you have questions and haven't seen or met these people, ask for them. Your nurse will message them to come see you. Speak up, and don't leave that building before you're prepared for the hours and days ahead. You need to understand your role in how you recover so you don't end up right back where you started. Do you know what medicines were prescribed? Were they sent to a pharmacy electronically, or were they printed? Who should you call if you have a problem or complication? Does your PCP know about your hospitalization? Ask the questions so there is a clear understanding between you and the system. Communication breakdown happens far more often than the hospital systems would ever want to admit. Don't leave the hospital until you understand what you (the patient) or you (the caregiver) should be doing.

What if you feel like you're being pushed out the door too soon? This happens all the time, but patients and family members don't say anything about it. They don't know that they can refuse to comply or they require clarification on issues. I want to bring up two terms that are like shields against the hospital suits that think of you as dollars and cents; "medically necessary" and "safely."

Insurance companies currently dictate medical policy in the hospital, not the providers that care for patients. For example, let's say your father had a bad case of pneumonia, and he was hospitalized for care. There are guidelines and metrics that the insurance companies say they'll pay for. They might allocate one night in the hospital for that particular diagnosis code that your doctor punched into the EMR. That usually means they're not very interested in paying for a second night in the hospital, because the guidelines say "most people" should be out after that overnight stay.

Well, what if your dad isn't capable of "safely" going home yet? Maybe he's still sick and in need of specialized care. Maybe he lives alone, or there's no "consistent caregiver," another good term to remember. You can appeal the upcoming discharge, stating that an additional night in the hospital, or transfer to an appropriate facility, is "medically necessary." It gives you a fighting chance to get the charges covered by insurance. Remember, hospital administrators and insurance adjusters look at the numbers, the black and white. They don't treat patients or practice medicine. Nothing is black and white when you practice medicine.

As a provider, I feel patients and families are far too quiet during our interaction. They don't ask questions. Whether that's because they don't know what to ask, they're too afraid to ask it, or just blindly trust the whitecoat to deliver all the appropriate information on a silver platter. Then, as soon as they see the doctor exit the exam room, they're flooded with dozens of questions that weren't answered. This is what leads to the poor patient outcomes and patient dissatisfaction. Or, it's at least a part of the bigger problem.

That's a long-winded way to say this: ASK QUESTIONS. Bring a notepad, or ask for paper, and as the questions pop into your head, write them down. If you're the loved one or friend of the patient, do this for them. Put yourself in your shoes and ask, "What would I need to know if I were in their position?"

As I'm writing this, I can recall a patient I had just this week that was in pretty bad shape. He was breathing heavily, sweating, and genuinely sick. His wife pulled out a notepad filled with scribbles, notes, and other facts. Some text was highlighted, and some was deleted. When I stopped talking and updating them on his latest result, she began firing questions at me. I loved it. I knew that this patient was in great hands, because he had someone in his corner that was prepared and organized. When I handed them (i.e., her) his discharge paperwork, she began to mark it up, circling the medications, and highlighting the pharmacy where I sent medications. She was on top of the situation.

We're just scratching the surface here. I could probably write an entire book about the hospital "system" as a whole, but that's not the purpose of this particular book. Now let's introduce some of the key players in medicine: The providers, the staff, and the options you have as a patient on where and how to receive care.

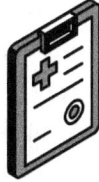

# CHAPTER 3
## WHERE DO I GO?

*Courage isn't about knowing the path, it's about taking the first step.*

–Katie Davis

I was almost finished with physician assistant school. The local hospital allowed me to pick up extra shifts in the ER to get training before I took my board exam. They would put me in the "fast track" area of the ER. Fast track is akin to being in an urgent care facility, but they charge ER fees. If you check into the ER with a "sore throat" as the main complaint, the front desk knows that you're probably not dying from that, so they designate you to the fast track.

I liked this role. As a very new provider (I'm still learning and shadowing people at this point), it was almost comforting knowing that the evening wouldn't be too stressful.

That's when this young couple walked in.

This couple was in their mid-20s, and you'd think they were walking into a restaurant or night club. They were dressed nicely and having a great time. They were laughing, holding onto each other and talking loudly while walking to their room. I didn't know which one was the patient. They certainly didn't look like they needed to be checked into the ER.

I walked in to gather their history and their chief complaint, i.e., their reason for coming to the ER at 11 pm on a Thursday. Still laughing, the entire interaction seemed to be like some big joke to them. It was hard for me not to smile and not let out a little chuckle as well. It seemed as though whatever led them to this point would end up being a good story one day.

"Hey everyone, I'm Arden. What brings y'all in tonight? The bar is across the street," I said, seeing as though they're comfortable enough with a little ribbing.

The girl, chuckling through her words, blurts out, "My boyfriend, um, well... he fell on something!" and they both explode with laughter.

"Fell on something, eh?" I replied, more perplexed than before.

He chimes in. "Yeah, we were playing around at her house when I found a drawer full of her toys." He holds his hands out in a parallel fashion as if he were measuring a fish he caught with his buddies. But he caught something else entirely.

"We were fooling around, and she said I should try it. So, I did." They were still laughing. "These people are quite amused with themselves," I thought to myself.

"So, let me get this straight," I asked. "I guess you came here because you couldn't get it out?"

"It gets better!" His partner said with exclamation. "There's more!"

He added, "Well, I was kind of into it. I wasn't ready for it to end. So I asked her to keep going."

I don't really know what to think or expect at this point. I'm trying to maintain some professionalism, but the circumstances are making that quite difficult. What else can this guy tell me?

I ask, "How long ago was it since you first inserted this device?"

"The first one? I don't know babe, what, maybe two hours ago?" he replied. My head almost rolled off my body.

"You mean to tell me that there are two things stuck in your rear end right now?"

"Three, actually." He said. His tone got a little more serious. His partner was still chuckling. "We think one still may still be vibrating," she said.

I did a quick exam and did hear a bit of humming from his abdomen. I certainly never heard that sound in someone's belly before, and I'll never forget it either. I quickly found my attending physician, gave him the rundown of what was in "fast track" and got the patient in a gown. I had already ordered the x-ray I wanted, and by the time I returned from my consultation with the physician, he was wheeled off to get the image taken.

When he got back, we reviewed the films. "Call the surgeon," the attending physician said. "He needs to see this right now."

The couple was in shock. "What do you mean? What are you calling the surgeon for? Can't you just take them out?"

"No sir," The doctor said, pointing to the images. "This one, right here? That's way up in there, and there's no way to get that out in here." The laughing couple went through numerous emotions in a matter of minutes.

What was very funny at first turned very serious in the blink of an eye. The gentleman ended up having a significant surgery that night. Everything turned out fine—and he and his partner still have quite a story to tell—but the situation could have turned badly very quickly.

While this is probably the most bizarre story I have to illustrate this topic, the truth is that patients go to the wrong place for care all the time. Yes, he was in the "Emergency Room," but the fast track area is designated for non-emergent conditions. He sat for hours waiting to be seen, not including the hours prior to arriving at the hospital. There was more than adequate time for the situation to go bad. In this chapter, I want to explain to you the key players in our healthcare system, show you their scope of practice, and allow you to determine when to use each of them.

Allow me to introduce you to the key players in the healthcare hierarchy–the medical staff.

The one you're likely most familiar with is the "physician." There are two types of medical doctors in the U.S. First are medical doctors (MDs) and the second are doctors of osteopathy (DOs). The difference is primarily in the training. DOs spend more time learning a "holistic approach" to medicine, whereas MDs have a more allopathic path to learning. Simply put, MDs are trained to use drugs, radiation, and/or surgery to treat disease,[7] and a DOs approach is more holistic, addressing the "whole person," including preventative healthcare and lifestyle modifications, to achieve healing in their patients.

As a patient, you'll notice a difference in their treatment styles, but it should be subtle. At the end of the day, both do an excellent job in their respective fields. The thing to remember is that the physician is who you're there to see. They are the one that will evaluate, diagnose, and treat your condition.

In today's world of medicine, there are other "providers" that offer patient care. If you didn't know any better, you'd say this was the "doctor" at the end of the interaction with you. I'm referring to physician associates/physician assistants (PAs) and advanced practice nurse practitioners (NPs). Both PAs and NPs provide a wide range of quality medical care. They work in primary care settings, ERs, in the operating room with surgeons, and in clinical research. They are held to rigorous standards in continuing education. The difference between a PA vs. an NP stems from their background and their training. PAs typically learn in a similar fashion to physicians, while NPs are taught to be "advanced nurses." Both are crucial to bringing quality medical care to a greater range of people. Again, as a patient, the intention is for you to not know or see a difference in the quality of care you receive.

After the providers, there are a sea of professionals who, in my opinion, don't get enough credit. I'm referring to the registered nurse (RN), licensed practical nurse (LPN) and licensed vocational nurse (LVN), as well as the many therapists, technicians, and other medical support staff who are truly the heroes in the healthcare community. These professionals do everything from take your blood pressure, draw your blood, dress your wounds, and perform many other tasks to keep the patient stable and well.

Regardless of where you visit, you will likely see all of these professionals in some capacity. The overwhelming majority of these people will properly introduce themselves and offer you their title (for me, it's required by law). If you don't know what they do or who they are, ask. They will be happy to tell you.

Now you know the "who," but what about the "where?" Where should I go when I get sick or injured?

For starters, let's talk about 911[8] What started off in 1957 as a number only to report fires, 911 became the universal "call for help" number in 1968, with the help of a partnership between the Federal Communications Commission (FCC) and the American Telephone and Telegraph Company (AT&T). The number was selected for its ease to remember, and that it was never used for an area code or service code. By the end of the 20th century, about 93% of the population was covered by some type of 911 service. Today, there are over 240 million calls to 911 each year.[9]

Can you begin to imagine the types of calls that 911 has to service? Not all are medical emergencies, and many aren't emergencies at all. I couldn't imagine answering that phone every day; I'll bet the operators hear some wild stories.

When is it appropriate to call 911 for a medical emergency?[10] Well, do you remember the emergencies discussed in Chapter 1? That's a great start. Facial drooping, slurred speech (signs of stroke), chest pain, shortness of breath, obvious bony deformity after a trauma; these are all great reasons to use the 911 public service. If there is a scenario where you are not comfortable determining what is an emergency and what isn't, by all means, call them. Often the highly trained operator can walk you through the situation and determine the next best steps. They may even send an ambulance to your location to have professionals take a look for themselves.

When is it not appropriate to call 911? Basically, anything that is not an immediate threat to life or limb. Tummy aches, scraped knees, and your cough that you have had for three weeks are all good examples.

What happens when you call 911?[11] Currently, you'd likely call from your cellphone. This means that the phone is not tied to a specific location. Most emergency calls from cellphones are routed to a central communications center. You may be talking to someone who is not familiar with your particular area. Someone will answer the call and state something along the lines of, "911, what is your emergency?" It is the caller's responsibility to act calmly and quickly, relaying important information in a clear, understandable tone. You need to include your name and precise location (e.g., cross-streets, landmarks, names of buildings, etc.), what the emergency is, and who needs help (e.g., name and age). Give them details, but keep it short. Tell them if the victim is breathing and if they're conscious. Then, *don't hang up*. The dispatcher will provide you with instructions on what to do while you're waiting for help to arrive.

My point is 911 is for life-threatening emergencies. This person in front of you is going to die or have significant morbidity if they're not treated, and fast. There have been cases where people have been charged with crimes for calling 911 for non-emergencies. For example, in 2015 a woman in Ohio called to complain about bad Chinese food and was charged with a misdemeanor.[12] Don't be like that woman.

If you call 911, they will expect you to have an emergency. So unless your complaint is so blatantly non-emergent, they will try to assist and send help in the form of EMS. There are three levels of EMS "technicians," i.e., basic, intermediate, and paramedic, each with varying degrees of training and ability. Once they arrive, they will assess the situation and determine the next best step for the safety of the patient. That could mean that they start administering medications through an IV (intravenous infusion of fluids and drugs), or they start life support and try to keep the patient alive. It all depends on the circumstances.

Something to remember when calling 911 for a transport to the hospital: It costs money.[13] The average transport in an ambulance is about $1,200. Remember, too, that if they perform services or administer medications while on the ride, you'll also be charged for that. So additional consideration must be understood when there's doubt on the emergent need of EMS care. Here are some other things to consider: Is your patient stable? Are they breathing, conversing, and able to move under their own power? Would a car ride be safe for them? How far away is the nearest hospital? While that rural family might have to wait upwards of 40 minutes for an ambulance, their commute to the hospital is only 10 minutes. All of this can play into that decision.

I want you to be prepared if 911 becomes an issue, so I'm including a free copy of my Emergency Action Plan (EAP) on my website.

## 1. Personal Information

| Full Name | Date of Birth | Gender |
|---|---|---|
| _____ | _____ | _____ |

| Address | Emergency Contact(s) | Primary Phone Number |
|---|---|---|
| _____ _____ | • Name: _____ <br> • Relationship: _____ <br> • Phone Number: _____ | _____ |

## 2. Medical History

| Chronic Conditions (e.g., diabetes, hypertension) | Allergies: (medications, food, others) | Blood Type (if known) |
|---|---|---|
| _____ <br> _____ | _____ <br> _____ | _____ |

## 3. Previous Surgical History

| List of Surgeries: (Include name/type of surgery and approximate dates) | | |
|---|---|---|
| _____ | _____ | _____ |
| _____ | _____ | _____ |

## 4. Current Medications

| Name of Medication | Dosage | Frequency | Purpose (e.g., blood pressure, diabetes) |
|---|---|---|---|
| _____ | | | _____ |
| _____ | _____ | _____ | _____ |
| _____ | | | _____ |

## 5. Physician(s) and Healthcare Providers

| Primary Care Physician | Specialists: Type (e.g., Cardiologist), |
|---|---|
| • Name: _____ <br> • Contact Information: _____ | • Name: _____ <br> • Contact Information: _____ |

# WHERE DO I GO?

## 6. Local Hospitals and Medical Facilities

| Preferred Hospital | Alternate Hospital | Pharmacy |
|---|---|---|
| • Name: _____ | • Name: _____ | • Name: _____ |
| • Relationship: _____ | • Relationship: _____ | • Relationship: _____ |
| • Phone Number: _____ | • Phone Number: _____ | • Phone Number: _____ |

## 7. Health Insurance Information

| Provider Name | Policy Number | Group Number (if applicable) | Contact Number for Verification |
|---|---|---|---|
| _____ | _____ | _____ | _____ |

## 8. Advanced Directives

| Resuscitation Preferences (CPR/DNR) | Living Will (brief summary and where to find the full document) | Healthcare Power of Attorney (contact information if different from emergency contact) |
|---|---|---|
| _____ <br> _____ | _____ <br> _____ <br> _____ <br> _____ | _____ |

## 9. Miscellaneous Information

| Language Preference | Special Instructions (e.g., pacemaker, hearing aids, disabilities | Religious Considerations (if relevant to medical care) |
|---|---|---|
| _____ | _____ <br> _____ <br> _____ | _____ <br> _____ <br> _____ |

## 10. Consent Statement for Emergency Use

I,........................................................ hereby authorize any emergency medical personnel, first responders, or healthcare providers to use the information provided in this document for the purposes of medical treatment and emergency care. This document is intended to communicate my medical history, current medications, healthcare preferences, and contact information for my primary care and emergency contacts in situations where I am unable to communicate for myself. I understand that this document contains sensitive personal health information and it is my responsibility to ensure its accuracy and safekeeping. I agree to update this information regularly to reflect any changes in my medical condition, treatment preferences, or emergency contacts.

This consent is given voluntarily and without coercion. I understand that I have the right to revoke this consent at any time, except to the extent that action has been taken in reliance on it.

Signature: _____

Date: _____

This document is key for your family to stay organized in the event of an emergency. All family members should be familiar with where it's stored and what it says/means. The downloadable copy can be found here: thehomemademd.com/eap

Ok, enough about emergencies. Most of the time, we're trying to figure out what to do with our non-emergent situation. Who should we go see, and who is going to be there when we go.

When it comes to selecting a medical facility to use, we are so fortunate to have a plethora of selections. Think about it: Today, there are pharmacies, urgent care clinics and doctor's offices seemingly on every corner. While some people in other parts of the world have to travel great distances to get any sort of medical care, ours is literally at our fingertips. I'll touch on telemedicine shortly.

Practically speaking, the decision largely depends on your needs and the amount of time you have. Are you looking for your checkup that you get once a year? Do you have a cold and have a critical work presentation on Friday? Do you have a bone protruding in the wrong direction? These three scenarios warrant different approaches.

The first scenario, that is, getting your checkup, is a job for your PCP. Traditionally, this would be a family practice trained physician, but PAs and NPs are assisting in this capacity also. PCPs are critical in the healthcare ecosystem and play a key role in keeping the ebbs and flows moving in the right direction.

The PCP sees their patients at least once a year. In fact, your "yearly checkup" is covered by most insurance plans at no out-of-pocket costs to you. If this is all you need with your doctor, great. This visit is just to keep an eye out for anything suspicious and make sure you're staying in good health. Often this visit could include blood draws for laboratory studies, injections/vaccinations, or scheduling procedures that are due at certain ages such as a mammography or colonoscopy.

PCPs also fill and refill certain medications that you may require. They manage common medical diagnoses like hypertension, diabetes, high cholesterol, and many other common issues that may require daily medication.

As you can imagine, you will develop a good relationship with this provider. And you should. You will see them at least once per year, perhaps more, and it's their job to ensure your health is trending in the right direction. It's important to have a PCP that you can trust and to whom you can speak frankly. They don't have time to guess at what's bothering you, and you don't want to waste your time and visit. As you can imagine, the PCP has a pretty busy schedule. A PCP typically will receive 30- and 60-minute blocks of time for their patients. At some bigger hospitals, they may cut that to 15/30 minute blocks. Even at the busiest possible schedule, that leaves only 32 people that one provider could see in an eight-hour day. With hundreds or even thousands of people in line to see that provider, it could take weeks to get on the schedule.

This obviously becomes a problem for most people who don't consider calling three weeks in advance for their sudden medical problem. While some providers leave a slot or two open for "sick visits," the COVID-19 pandemic has changed how many PCPs see patients. There are many PCPs, even some entire hospital systems, that will not see sick patients. If you call your provider's office right now, and you tell them you're sick, they might not offer you a slot. Rather, they may send you to the nearest urgent care or ER for care. This is obviously something you should be aware of and be prepared for. I'll discuss more on urgent care shortly.

ERs are designed for emergencies in mind. If your life or limb is in danger, the ER is the place to be. Providers are specifically trained to work in the ER when minutes and seconds could mean the difference between life and death. The medicine is quality, but the experience can sometimes be a bit chaotic. Think for a second what stress you would be under if it's 3 am and you just finished performing chest compressions on a "lifeless" patient. After what seemed to take hours, the patient is stabilized. You have a quick celebration, but then you have to see the next patient in line. Can you imagine what it takes to switch gears and walk into the next room, all but completely forgetting the previous patient's situation? It's amazing what these people do on a daily basis. It's also very hard work, and it takes a toll on them physically and mentally. With the shortest life expectancy among their peers[14], and a suicide rate more than twice that of the general population[15], the stress is overwhelming. I mention this to remind you that if you're in the ER, it's a stressful place, for you and the provider. Approach the situation calmly and logically to achieve the best results.

I also want to mention specialists. Doctors don't stop after they complete medical school. Most, if not all, continue on to a residency program where they specialize in something other than general medicine. This residency program can be as short as three years for your primary care specialties and as many as seven or more in your surgical specialties.

Personally, I don't think you should be scheduling with specialists unless you know your problem is in need of specialist care. For example, you don't need a pulmonologist to see you for your cough for three weeks. You don't need to see a gastroenterologist for your two days of upset stomach. You don't need an oncologist because you have this bump on your leg.

My request is to learn the system, understand how it works, then use it to your advantage. Is that to say that there are no reasons whatsoever to schedule an appointment with a specialist before talking to anyone else? No. There are no black and white situations in medicine. But your PCP is likely a much better place to start. You could also go to urgent care.

Urgent care is a great addition to our medical landscape[16], and I've grown to respect the concept of the specialty. What started in the 1970s as a means to assist smaller communities receive more quality healthcare, the specialty has grown to include close to 10,000[17] urgent care facilities by 2019. Urgent care facilities are usually easily accessible

WHERE DO I GO?

in a commercial building near your favorite coffee shop or clothing store. The wait times are typically far less than an ER, the care is excellent, and the cost is extremely affordable compared to their ER counterparts. Urgent care can be a quick solution for many problems that arise on a daily basis, and the visit can keep you out of the ER. It's estimated that 27% of ER visits could have been effectively handled by an urgent care or retail clinic. That would save 4.4 billion dollars per year!

The biggest issue with urgent care, depending on who you ask, is the limitations in their scope of practice. They usually cannot order many laboratory tests or advanced imaging, although many urgent care facilities can perform x-rays. This leads to confusion and frustration for patients who have waited for care, only to be turned away and not receiving the answers or sufficient care they require. This happens to me personally once or twice per shift.

Time is also against the provider while in urgent care. While PCPs and specialists can schedule their visits, urgent care providers have to deal with every condition that walks in their door. Imagine if you had 100 patients to see in a 12-hour shift. That gives the provider and staff seven minutes and 12 seconds to check the patient in, triage them, obtain their vital signs and a brief history, have the provider see and evaluate the patient, order any pertinent tests, Note that some tests take 15 minutes to run, document the visit, write prescriptions, print paperwork, and discharge the patient. Providers and staff do not have time to eat, go to the bathroom, take a phone call, or write an email. And since there is an increased demand for testing and a decrease in providers seeing their own patients, urgent care facilities are inundated with days like this.

For the patient, this means that you're going to see your provider for a limited amount of time. If you come into a busy urgent care expecting to sit and chat with your provider for 30 minutes, you'll likely leave disappointed. As a provider, I take pride in my ability to connect with patients quickly and achieve this connection promptly, but I still realize that visits are too short. While unfortunate, it's unavoidable if I intend to see all 100 patients before our doors close.

While 27% of ER visits could be handled by urgent care, I'll bet that many more urgent care visits could be handled at home, and that's precisely why I'm writing this book. Section 2 will have more tips and tricks on treating yourself at home.

Telemedicine is another healthcare alternative. Since the COVID-19 pandemic, we had to get creative in how we saw patients. Telemedicine has been around prior to the pandemic, but the pandemic escalated its use out of sheer necessity. Prior to 2020, telemedicine was a fringe addition to a few clinics, and used only in extreme circumstances. But we as a community have grown to embrace it. We realized that there are groups of people who can be served very well with the addition of this technology, and with the invention of accessories the patient can use at home, providers can see what they'd normally see in the clinic.

There is certainly a place for telemedicine in our healthcare ecosystem, and I fully encourage you to take advantage of it if and when it's offered. Understand one thing: As I mentioned about urgent care facilities being limited with regard to what they can do and treat safely, telemedicine's scope of practice will be even further restricted. Don't expect to get 100% of your medical needs met by some doctor on your mobile phone screen. We're still pretty limited in that area, but at the rate healthcare is evolving, don't be surprised if that's the case in the near future.

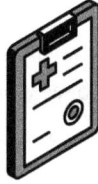

# CHAPTER 4
## Prepare For Your Visit

*Good luck is when opportunity meets preparation, while bad luck is when lack of preparation meets reality*

—Eliyahu Goldratt

"She's balling her eyes out," my nurse told me as I walked out of another patient room. "I can't console her, and I can't understand what has her so upset."

I'm working a string of long shifts in urgent care, and it's getting to be the end of my shift. I'm starting to think about my relaxing three-day "weekend" in the middle of the week, when this patient storms into urgent care. My front desk staff brought her back very quickly, as they thought something was terribly wrong once they saw her. She was clearly disheveled, wearing pajama pants and a baggy sweatshirt with flip flops, hair out of place, and makeup smearing from the tears rolling down her cheeks.

"Ma'am, what has you so upset?" I ask as I enter the room. I brought one of my coworkers with me, just in case there was some type of sensitive issue that needed to be addressed.

"I-I... I just can't believe this is happening to me!" More tears. Other patients are opening their doors to see what is causing all the commotion.

"Ma'am, we're here to help you, but I need to know what's going on." She responded, through tears, "My life is over. I don't know what to do."

I was genuinely confused, and so was my coworker. "What do you mean?" I ask.

"Well, I've had this cough for like a week, and I've lost a few pounds. So when I saw this spot on my neck...." She lifted away the sweatshirt to show me this tiny little abscess, only slightly larger than a pimple you'd find on your face. "I started to look up what all that could mean."

"Okay. Is that what got you all upset?" I say cautiously.

"Well yes! Don't you understand? This is cancer!" She again bursts into tears.

It took several minutes to calm her down. This poor woman was so upset from what Dr. Google told her that she could not function. She was completely paralyzed with fear.

About 30 minutes and one popped abscess later, the patient was much more at ease. I spent a good deal of time over the next hour or so telling her what I'm about to tell you here. She left urgent care that night with much more knowledge about medically caring for yourself, and I hope you do too.

I never want to come across as some all-knowing, obnoxious provider that can't appreciate someone being an advocate for their own health. I think there are many providers and staff that would have treated that patient I mentioned previously very poorly because "she Googled her symptoms." Well guess what: I know that *all of you* probably Google your symptoms. Is that a bad thing? Not necessarily. Googling your symptoms and taking that six-year old blog post you found as solid medical advice is a terrible idea. It always will be. It's incredibly easy to find a wealth of information online regarding your particular circumstances, and you can get an extensive amount of sound information in your search. But if you don't understand the human body, if you don't understand the pathophysiology of diseases and how your immune system works and what drugs do when you take them, I think you're asking for trouble.

Does that mean you need to know all that information? Of course not. That's why we, as professionals, went to school. We get paid to share that knowledge with our patients. But one way to score huge with your provider is to come to the visit prepared. I encourage all of you to Google your symptoms. Google away! I want you to learn as much as you want about your particular circumstances. And once you obtain all that research and new knowledge, I want you to compile it and organize your thoughts, and I want you to come to your provider to have a discussion about it. There's no provider on Earth that would ignore you for being prepared to speak intelligently about your particular situation, not a good one anyway. Instead of taking your research as doctrine for your condition, use it as a talking point with your provider. It'll help you understand where you stand, and it'll indicate to your provider that you are taking your situation seriously.

If you're going to Google your symptoms, there are several websites that you can use. Symptomate.com[18] uses Artificial Intelligence (AI), doctors' knowledge, literature, and statistical data gathered from thousands of patient cases to give you recommendations on the state of your health. You add your symptoms, and the app will give you a recommendation. Medscape, Pubmed, WebMD and others are good resources as well.

Again, I wouldn't take this as gospel, but it's a tool–and a fairly good one–especially if you have a limited background in medicine. At the end of the day, I think it's beneficial to possess knowledge, but communication with your provider still trumps a search for online medical information.

Let's say you made an appointment with your provider. Before you arrive, ask the office if there is any paperwork you need to complete beforehand. They'll email you the packet and help you get started. This saves you time, saves the office time, and helps your provider understand what they're dealing with behind that exam room door. Bring your document that you received from this book and give it to them, or use it as a reference when you're filling out your paperwork. Double check your wallet or purse and make sure you have an ID and your insurance information.

And now, the visit. Take a minute to put yourself in the position of your provider. Depending on what kind of treatment you're receiving (e.g., urgent care, primary care, emergent care, etc.), you're likely to have a very finite amount of time with this provider. In the case of urgent care and the ER, this could literally be a matter of minutes. Providers have been trained, both during their schooling and by their respective employers, to see people incredibly quickly. Big hospital systems actually invest time and money into learning what providers can do or say in the exam room to give the perception that the provider spent more time in the room than the patient realizes. In other words, they learn ways to make a three-minute visit feel like a 10-minute visit. They will sit down, make eye contact, ask very specific but open-ended questions to make you elaborate. By talking about yourself, you experience a sense of connection to the person asking the questions. This gives you the impression that it took more time to make this connection, and since you spent more time with the provider, you feel more understood.

This might feel a bit deceptive, but I still believe that the provider has good intentions. In my practice, I feel as if I am still genuine with these connections that I make. Are some of my visits short? You bet! They have to be short if I am to see 80-plus patients in one day. My point in telling you this is simple: Now that you are equipped with this information, you have the ability to control the length of the visit. You may not require more time, but if you do, you have the power. With the research you compiled prior to the visit, you can ask appropriate and relevant questions. Ask the provider to elaborate on their diagnosis. Ask how you can prevent this from happening again, or what you should do to prevent the symptoms from getting worse. If you've done research, you'll have questions. In fact, most of my patients have tons of questions without one second of research, but most people are too afraid to ask them. Once that provider leaves your room, there's no guarantee they're coming back. Keep them in the room until you are satisfied with the information you need.

So you've met with your provider, you discussed your research and are open minded to hear what the provider has to say. If I were there, I'd be handing you a medal. But what do you do with the information they just gave you?

First, I want you to update your list. Is it on your Google drive like I suggested? Get that phone out and update it to keep the most up-to-date information. This is especially important if the provider prescribed new meds. Were you diagnosed with high blood pressure and started a new medication? Get the medicine name, the dosage, the time you're supposed to take it, and how many refills you have. Put all that information in your spreadsheet to keep track.

As a provider, when a patient can't remember what medication(s) they're taking, it limits me and how effective I can be to treat you that day. I can't tell you how many times people tell me, "oh, it's the round blue pill." That doesn't help me in the slightest. The metoprolol 10 milligram tablet at your local pharmacy could look like 45 other medications on the market. Plus, it's just not a safe way to tell a provider what medication you're on. Medications can be identified in certain programs and apps by their color, shape, and the numbers and letters that are scored on them. This is good for a last minute, need-to-know situation, but since you're reading this book, you have plenty of time to prepare.

45

One of the questions I get most frequently revolves around taking medicine when you don't feel bad. "Why do I have to take this blood pressure/diabetes medicine when I feel completely fine?" They'll ask me this question upon receiving their prescriptions. It's important to ask these questions when you're sitting in front of your provider, but I'll tell you that there are several medical conditions that have no symptoms until they become a major problem. Consider your car, for example. When you purchase a car, you understand that car ownership comes with certain responsibilities, maintenance being a primary one. For example, if you don't keep oil fresh in the car, bad things can happen. While few of us have actually observed what results occur when a car runs on tainted oil, we still know that unfortunate outcomes are inevitable if the car doesn't receive an oil change.

Here's the thing: The car won't give you some big warning signs that it's about to blow up; it just blows up. You may get a warning light to tell you it's time to change the oil, sure. But the car won't start talking to you and tell you that its engine is about to seize.

Many of these medical conditions work the exact same way. High blood pressure typically doesn't hurt. Rather, prolonged high blood pressure can lead to severe, and even fatal, conditions.

Since we're discussing preparation regarding your health, you're never too young to assign a healthcare power of attorney[19] and have a will drafted. A healthcare power of attorney (HCPA) is an individual that you designate to make medical decisions on your behalf. This is usually your spouse or significant other, or it can be anyone you designate through this document. You obviously want to trust this person, as they could be responsible for life-and-death decisions for you. When I had my appendix removed, my wife was able to answer for me since she is my HCPA.

A will is a legal document[20] that explains your wishes regarding property or minor children you may have. If you don't have a will, distribution of these items could be left to a court system, resulting in lost time, money, and heartache for your loved ones.

I'm not an attorney, but I have both of these documents for myself and for my wife in a fireproof safe in my house. And I encourage my patients to have one as well. It  simply provides additional comfort knowing that things are set up the way I'd like them to be.

After a visit with any medical provider, the next stop is usually to your local pharmacy. To one that doesn't understand medicine, this place can be equally as confusing as the doctor's office. I don't want that for you, so I'm going to go over some tricks to make the trip to the pharmacy just as easy.

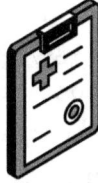

# CHAPTER 5

## Navigating Your Pharmacy

*Being a caregiver requires infinite patience, physical and emotional strength, health care navigation skills, and a sense of humor, which can be hard to come by after sleepless nights and demanding days.*

–Rosalynn Carter

Retail pharmacies are huge moneymakers. The estimated market size for 2022 is $346 billion. [21]There are roughly 60,000 pharmacies in the U.S.[22] Two-thirds of those are one of the top five "big box" pharmacies like CVS, Walgreens, or Walmart. Wherever you're reading this, you are likely to know just how far the nearest pill box is located. You can probably even walk there. You may have even purchased this book from one. These big box pharmacies fight for real estate all over the U.S. It's funny how they always seem to land right across the street from each other.

Retail medicine has not escaped the corporate takeover of America. Only about 6% of U.S. pharmacies are considered "independent."[23] This is a disservice, especially to our more rural areas and our under-served communities, as these communities typically rely on independent owners for their medications. Since the corporate mass retailers are able to offer drugs at an incredibly low price–sometimes even at a loss–to attract business. The independent guys aren't able to compete.

The big guys aren't all bad, however, and while they're busy driving prices down, a new player has emerged and proliferated during the COVID-19 pandemic. The online retail pharmacy is rapidly becoming a key component to the marketplace. People are ordering their medications online and they'll be delivered to their doorstep. Providers are able to electronically send medications to these pharmacies, making it even easier for the patient.

My biggest complaints with the current state of the retail pharmacy industry include two main topics. First, the overwhelmingly complex and confusing pricing of medications, and second, the lack of transparency of pricing to the consumer.

While researching for this book, I was amazed to see how complicated the pricing process is for retail and specialty pharmacies. Drug stores get their medications either directly from the manufacturer or from a wholesaler. The stores are usually contracted with, and reimbursed by, pharmacy benefit managers (PBMs). PBMs create formularies, negotiate rebates (i.e., discounts paid by a drug manufacturer to a PBM) with manufacturers, process claims, create pharmacy networks, review drug utilization, and occasionally manage mail-order specialty pharmacies.[24] So when you go to collect your new prescription with your health insurance, the price should have been predetermined, based on the formulary for your particular insurance. You pay your copay, and the insurance company pays the rest.

But this is where it gets entirely too confusing.

The wholesale cost to each pharmacy could vary, often significantly. This cost difference could depend on whether the drug is generic or brand name (I'll discuss this in a minute), how much market power the pharmacy has, and what types of benchmarks have been established.

The wholesalers—and there are only three of them in the U.S.—mark up the drug, sell it to the pharmacy, then the pharmacy gets reimbursed on the back end with private insurance or Medicaid. This is how the little guy gets squeezed out. The big boxes can command a much cheaper price for a drug since it will be offered in thousands of stores across the country, while the little guy is usually working with a small number of prescriptions or locations.

Enter mail order and e-commerce pharmacies. Initially, this was a bit controversial, as most mail order companies were/are owned by PBMs. This means that as the PBMs create your formulary, they can incentivize the end-user to use their mail order option in lieu of using the cheapest and/or most appropriate medication.

I personally despise entities and organizations meddling in the delicate relationship that is the patient and provider. Why are insurance companies and these PBMs dictating *your* healthcare? It's not uncommon for people not to fill medications because the they are too expensive. This company can look like a savior when they offer an alternative medicine at a discount. But is this what's best for the patient? This situation is the ugly side of medicine. The fix is even more complicated, but I hope we start with making prices more transparent to the end-users prior to the point of sale. You should be able to know exactly what your medicine will cost before you leave your provider's office.

The e-pharmacies are getting pretty good at this. There are even companies like GoodRx that will display a pretty accurate cost of a particular medicine at your pharmacy and the ones nearby. For me and my family, this has been incredibly helpful in selecting certain medications, as the prices can vary so drastically. E-pharmacies will be interesting to watch as more players get involved, especially companies that don't have current ties to big pharma.

I'll give you a personal example of the pricing craziness. My wife and I take one medication, same drug, same dose. We use a local big box pharmacy because it is on our way home, and because my employer-sponsored healthcare plan is contracted with this particular store. In the past six months, we have never paid the same price twice. There have been times where we pay two different prices during the same visit. The lowest the medication has been was around $27, and the highest was $92. Astonishing, right? I understand that this is one instance, but my patients tell me all the time that they cannot afford the medication that I prescribed, and we need to devise another option.

Since you and I can't control the disparity that is the cost of retail prescription drugs by reading this book, let's focus on something we *can* control: Over the counter (OTC) medications.

Remember me telling you that many big box and retail companies will undersell their generic drugs? They do that for a reason: They want you to shop at their stores. Your neighborhood pharmacy makes about 60% of their revenue with the sale of your medications, but they make almost 40% of their revenue through retail sales. They bank on you arriving, getting your drugs at the pharmacy, which is usually in the back of the store, allowing you to walk past all the goodies, and selecting a few things on the way out. So while they know they will make a good chunk from your drug purchase, they bank on you picking up milk and a magazine on your way out.

I'm not bashing the business model. In fact, it's genius; that's why CVS and Walgreens are on every suburban corner on Earth. That's what it feels like, right? I tell you this so you can be prepared when you walk in. You are being seduced.

I'm writing this book to give awareness to those who may be a bit clueless as to how the healthcare system works. I want to also provide you with some practical advice on what you can safely do at home to make yourself feel better. With regards to western medicine and medications, here's some information on how to stock your home medicine cabinet.

Remember, I don't know you, and I'm not your provider. So always check your own allergies, take medications as directed on the label, and consult with your medical provider before going rogue.

The first thing I'd consider for my medicine cabinet would be pain-relieving medications. Medications like acetaminophen (Tylenol®) and ibuprofen (Motrin®) are my go-to recommendations. I typically tell my patients to alternate these medications, taking one or the other every three hours. Taking these medications like this seems to offer a synergistic effect, meaning they're more helpful together than they are by themselves.

While the OTC doses for ibuprofen and acetaminophen are 400 milligrams and 325-650 milligrams, respectively, the prescription doses are 800 milligrams for ibuprofen and 1,000 milligrams for acetaminophen, each taken every six hours.

See what I just said there? When your provider prescribes you ibuprofen, it's usually 600 milligrams or 800 millgrams. This is the exactly the same as taking three or four OTC pills of the same medication. Why pay for a prescription when you have the same medication at home in your cabinet?

Now, I don't like acetaminophen for kids, and I don't like it for pregnant women. My guess is, with a little research, you'll understand why.

Number two on the list would be some sort of allergy medication. There are four main OTC allergy medications: Zyrtec®, Allegra®, Claritin® and Xyzal®. Some allergy medications are combined with a "D" variety that includes a decongestant called pseudoephedrine. Sudafed® is a medication can be purchased separately or in combination with an allergy medicine. This medicine is "behind the counter," meaning, it's behind the pharmacy counter but does not require a prescription. In order to purchase this medication, you'll need to show identification to the staff; they want to make sure you don't have a knack for preparing meth in your kitchen.

"Well, Arden, which one should I get?" That's the million dollar question. In my professional opinion, one of these medications is likely going to work better for you than the others. I tell my patients to go buy a small package of the one you want to try first. Try the entire package, and document your experience. Compare your experience and the extent of your symptom relief. The one that best suited you, wins.

I also believe that not everyone needs the Sudafed® that resides behind the pharmacy counter. The decongestant works well, but it is not without its side effects. The medication is excitatory in nature, which means that everything "ramps up." Your heart rate and blood pressure will increase, and you may feel a bit jittery and nervous. Some people with established heart conditions or high blood pressure should just pass on this medication. If that's not you, feel free to add it to your pharmacy cabinet.

Another allergy medicine is Benadryl®, or diphenhydramine. I always chuckle when I'm walking down pharmacy aisles and read the labels of certain medications. Companies will market medications for more than one indication. While we may recognize Benadryl® as an allergy medicine because it makes you sleepy, it's commonly sold as a sleep aid. It's not my choice of a sleep aid, but it's important to mention. Always read the labels before you buy medications. Know what you're buying and what you're putting into your body.

So you can use Benadryl® for mild allergic reactions and seasonal allergies, but remember; it will likely make you a bit drowsy.

While we're mentioning allergic reactions, steroid creams are important to keep handy for those itchy and scratchy bumps and rashes that you may occasionally experience. You want to have a steroid and/or Benadryl® cream to help with mild allergic reactions. We don't use steroid creams near the eyes or in sensitive areas, like the crotch, because it can pull the pigment out of your skin. If you feel the need to use these creams for longer than a week, get someone to look closely at your situation. We want to be sure we're not treating you inappropriately.

Stomach and gastrointestinal (GI) issues offer several OTC medications. There's usually an entire aisle dedicated to this problem. If you require GI meds in the house, here's what I recommend.

I love Pepto Bismol® as a good go-to upset stomach medication. It's one of the first medications I recommend in the clinic to patients with an upset stomach, nausea, and "just not feeling well." Imodium® (loperamide) is good also, but if I had to pick one, it'd be Pepto. In addition, Tums® are good antacid tablets to use for occasional heartburn.

I treat all my constipation patients with OTC medications. There are three constipation medications I'd keep at home: Miralax®, magnesium citrate, and Dulcolax® suppositories. I treat constipation with those medicines in that order. On day one of constipation, I recommend Miralax® in the morning, followed by a second dose in the early afternoon. Don't take these medicines right before bed, unless you want a date with your toilet that night.

On the second day, I recommend half of the bottle of magnesium citrate. They come flavored now, but they're not very tasty. However, they work really well. Usually those two medicines do the trick. If not—and you need a little extra help—it's time for the suppository. I've never had a patient have the need to go beyond step three. I am not saying it doesn't happen, so if it does in your case, you may need to see a doctor.

To stop diarrhea, Imodium® or Pepto Bismol® are your OTC medicines. GI bugs usually hit hard and fast, and if you find yourself using these medications for longer than three- to five days, it may be time to get checked out by a professional. As with any case of the runs, you *must* remain hydrated. I don't really care if you don't eat for a few days. Remember the Rule of Three: Humans can go about three minutes without air, three days without water, and three weeks without food. Replenish those fluids!

Water is still the gold standard when it comes to liquid replenishment. There are myriad products out there that will lure you into thinking "you need this," and "you're deficient in that," but overall, water is king. I have come to appreciate the science behind electrolyte supplementation in your water, particularly when a deficiency is expected, e.g., you're sick, or you've been working out really hard.

I like a product called "LMNT."[25] This product consists of powdered electrolytes in a package the size of a sugar pack. The only three ingredients are sodium, potassium and magnesium. If you experience headaches, mental fog or muscle cramps throughout the day or after intense exercise, LMNT will all but eliminate them. LMNT is now readily available and very portable. You add the powder into your water and you're ready to go. If you look at the ingredients, you'll realize that it'll taste a bit salty. That's the idea. Check out drinklmnt.com to pick some up.

There are a few items that aren't OTC that I would still recommend adding to your medicine cabinet. It may be as easy as having a discussion with your PCP to obtain them, or you can consider a telemedicine appointment to obtain the prescription. These are items that I'd rather have and not need, than need and not have.

The first item is an EpiPen®. Especially if you have children, or if you have a known severe allergy, this should be easy to obtain. They have a long shelf life, and even if it's expired, an old Epipen® is better than dying from anaphylaxis.

The second item would be Bactroban® ointment, also known as mupirocin. While I don't recommend ointment use regularly for common scrapes and burns, mupirocin can treat common skin conditions like impetigo and mild skin abscesses usually caused by staph infections. The pharmacy will suggest their triple antibiotic ointment, but there have been studies that demonstrate ointments like Neosporin® are practically useless. In some cases, the use of these ointments can actually lead to an increased risk of infection.[26]

Silvadene® cream (SSD) is a burn ointment/lotion that used to be my personal, first-line treatment for burns that presented in my clinic. But as time passes, and more literature is published, treatment protocols change. Today we know that something as simple as unprocessed honey can be a better treatment for mild burns than the expensive prescription SSD. Hydrocolloid dressings, also known as DuoDERM®, are flexible bandages used to treat minor burns. When compared to SSD, these wounds "healed faster, showed better appearance after healing and better repigmentation, required fewer and less elaborate dressing changes, and were less costly to treat."[27]

This is great news, as both of these items are available everywhere and are very inexpensive. One of them even makes a great addition to toast.

Last on this list would be a stockpile of medications you need to take on a regular (or emergent) basis.[28] If you are taking any long-term prescriptions, running out and not being able to get them would be a huge problem. The world is a fragile place, and if pharmacies shut down, you could be in for some trouble. Enter Jasemedical.com. This company was founded to provide people the means to get surplus medications, antibiotics and other prescription items as a personal medication emergency kit. Be prepared. (If you consider purchasing, use my code "JAM-1687" for 10% off your order.)

To complete your medicine cabinet contents, I like to keep a variety of bandages, splints, and wraps for scrapes and orthopedic issues. I also like to keep lip balm, vapor rub, lotions, and sinus rinse accessories like distilled water and salt packets.

If you're looking for an all-in-one option, there are products on the market that sell everything you'd need in a nice portable back or pack. I personally use and recommend MyMedic for all my portable kit needs, but they sell products that could serve as a great home medical kit as well.

I've mentioned several OTC medications, but I didn't touch on any one in particular. That would require its own a book.

I want to summarize the last few pages in the following bullet points:

- Read the label. There are many marketing dollars spent to make you spend more than you possibly need.

- Understand "brand name" vs. "generic" drugs and what that means for your body.
- Understand what's a "side effect" and what's an "allergy" to a medication or product.
- If it's a supplement or an herb, it's not regulated by anyone, and therefore could be anything. Do your research, and tread cautiously.

If all else fails, and you still feel a bit confused, talk to the pharmacist. They will discuss your options with you and offer their knowledge for you to make the best decision.

When it comes to paying for a medication — especially a prescription medicine — don't be afraid to put your negotiation skills to the test. As I mentioned with my personal medications and the price differences, ask the pharmacist or pharmacy staff to see what options you have available to get the costs reduced. There are several programs available today, such as GoodRx, for example, that will contract prices with drugs and pharmacies. These prices typically beat my own contracted price through my insurance. Sure, the money doesn't go towards my deductible, but my deductible is so high that it doesn't really concern me. Consider all options, and make the best decision for you and those involved.

I can write forever on medications alone. Since I have been trained in the western medicine approach, i.e., find a diagnosis, throw medicine at it, repeat, I have spent much of my education on learning drugs, their intended use, and their side effects. That said, humanity got this far without most of this them. There are certainly times where medications are required, and thank God we have them. The rest of the time, good health is achieved in spite of the medications upon which we rely. To avoid this entire chapter, eat a healthy, anti-inflammatory diet, get appropriate sleep, have systems in place to cope with stress, and avoid as much exogenous stress as often as possible, and pray you have some good genetics.

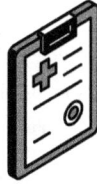

# CHAPTER 6
## How Insurance Works

*He who has health, has hope; and he who has hope, has everything.*

–Thomas Carlyle

The Center for Disease Control (CDC) says 31.6 million people were uninsured in 2020. The rest of us are left wondering what our insurance policy actually offers or covers. There is so much confusion surrounding insurance that it baffles most insurance employees. Imagine how the typical American feels.

The fact is that insurance plans are like fingerprints. They're all different, they all have particulars, nuances, and challenges. Some plans only want you to see certain providers. Some plans come with free health club benefits. Some plans will pay for all your medical services, while some won't pay anything until you reach your deductible. Confused yet? Allow me to shed some light on insurance for you.

I'm going to start with the basics, and can take it from there. First, there are two major types of insurance providers: The public sector, (i.e., government sponsored plans such as Medicare and Medicaid), and the private sector offered by private insurance companies. They branch off from there, and with the Affordable Care Act (ACA), there's a little crossover.

There are Health Maintenance Organizations (HMOs) and Preferred Provider Organizations (PPOs) in the private world. HMOs give you a set list of providers you can see, and that's it. If you see someone not on the list, your insurance does not cover the appointment, although there are likely exceptions in the case of emergencies. You also have to see your PCP first before seeing a specialist. So if you break a bone, your family doctor has to refer you to an orthopedist for care.

A PPO is a little more complicated, a little more expensive, but a little easier to see the provider you wish. A PPO also has a list of preferred providers, called "in-network," where you get the most benefits. If you choose to see "out-of-network" providers, you'll still be covered, but you're probably going to be penalized with a higher deductible, higher copay, and less coverage. It's still a choice. You also don't have to see your PCP first; rather, you can make an appointment with a specialist and bypass the PCP if needed.

Most people are enrolled in a PPO plan. So if you're confused, or if you don't know what kind of plan you have, you can bet it's a PPO.

Most of us are offered plans through our employer. In that case, we get little choice as to what that policy specifically offers. We mostly get to make few decisions as to how much we want to pay monthly, such as premiums, relative to the plans your employer offers. This employer-sponsored insurance plan helps keep our out-of-pocket costs down, as the employer and their insurance broker contracted and negotiated prices for that particular plan. If you were to try to buy the same plan on the private market, you'd likely pay a lot more for it.

Something to note about high-deductible plans; You're often eligible to open a Health Savings Account, or HSA, with high-deductible plans.[29] Think of it like a debit card for medical expenses. An HSA gives you the ability to put money away tax-free, thereby lowering your taxable income, use it for qualified expenses tax-free, and if you have an invested HSA, earn money tax-free.

This is different from the Flexible Spending Account (FSA) that began in the 1970s. That program is a yearly "use it or lose it" program. If you have money remaining at the end of the term, that money is forfeited. Imagine Billy Madison in the tub screaming, "HSAs are better!" That's how I remember it.

HSAs can be used for many medical expenses. From bandaids to tampons, prescriptions to eyeglasses, and your kids' orthotics. Even massages. I purchased all my MyMedic gear with my HSA card and placed the kits in my car as a mobile kit. Get an HSA. Your wallet will thank you.

Generally speaking, when we're searching for insurance plans, there are a couple of terms we're looking for. The first one is a deductible. That is what the insured person (or family) is financially responsible for prior to the insurance company coverage. In general, the higher your deductible, the cheaper the premium. There are such things as ultra-high deductible plans that are good primarily for emergency use. These plans are designed to keep you covered in case of an emergency, but otherwise you don't use it, or do not get a benefit from it.

Once your deductible is met, the insurance plan shares the cost with you, called coinsurance, or copay. This number can vary wildly and is usually printed on your insurance card. For some instances, the insurance would cover at 100% after your deductible. Some are 80/20, some are 70/30. The coinsurance could also vary, depending on the circumstances. You may be covered at 80% on medications, but only 50% on hospital stays. Again, plans are like fingerprints.

Insurance companies typically have a preferred network of providers and hospital groups that they work with. This is called in-network care. Everything will typically be cheaper in-network as opposed to out-of-network, but there are times when the policy will cover out-of-network costs, e.g., if your network doesn't have a particular specialty, or there's an emergency when you're out of town. Sometimes, out-of-network care won't count towards your deductible, or you'll have a separate column for out-of-pocket deductibles, which is typically higher than in-network.

Insurance policies will have insurance benefits. Usually, these policies will cover preventative care at 100%. This includes examinations such as your yearly evaluation with your provider, kids' wellness visits and shots, and some wellness screenings. Some policies include gym memberships, incentives for healthy living, such as not smoking, keeping a low BMI, being married etc., and access to programs and education to help you live a healthy lifestyle.

There are many other factors and criteria to consider when selecting an insurance plan, or even an employer for that matter, if you know about their insurance benefits beforehand. Knowing and understanding these concepts will get you started. Something to keep in mind, especially if you have an employee-sponsored healthcare plan, is to utilize the resources they already have prepared for you. If your employer went to the trouble to prepare a robust healthcare plan for you, they probably have a graph, booklet, or summary of the plan and what it offers you. Before you begin going through all the fine print and trying to decipher what's what, ask your employer for the benefits summary. It's usually well-organized and easy to read.

After every encounter where you use your insurance, you'll receive something called an Explanation of Benefits, or EOB. This document explains the breakdown of costs for your treatment and how the insurance plan was applied to your bill. It'll have an estimate as to what you're likely to owe, but it's not a bill. The bill will come from the service provider. I find that some insurances quickly submit these EOBs; others, not so much. I've often received EOBs months after the encounter, long after I've paid what I was asked to pay. What I now do is call my insurance provider prior to handing over any money. With cost transparency, these EOBs should be expedited. I'm not personally holding my breath.

This part gets really confusing.

My wife recently brought our oldest son to the hospital. I was out of town, and she was afraid something was wrong with him. She brought him to our ER. After a six-hour evaluation, he was able to return home safely.

A month later, we began receiving the bills. Three different ones for the same encounter, in fact. We received a bill for the hospital services, i.e.,nursing staff, sheets, gauze, etc., a bill for the doctor's services billed from a physician's group that contracts with the hospital to staff it, and a bill for the radiology group who read his x-ray. I did not receive the EOB in the mail prior to this, and I noticed the bill was extremely high for the services that were rendered.

That's when I started calling.

I probably spent 10 hours on the phone collectively among the groups and my insurance company. Ultimately, it was determined that the hospital collected my insurance information, but they never processed it for the encounter. So they were giving me a cash price for the visit, not the price after my insurance was applied.

A couple of weeks later, I received the adjusted bill. The bill was about 60% less than before, and the insurance company contribution was appropriately reflected on the bill.

If you take anything from this book, it should be this: **You have to be your own advocate, and you have to speak up for yourself.**

This means being willing to put in the time, communicate with the offices/hospitals where you were treated, **DOCUMENT EVERYTHING,** and take a deep breath. Something will undoubtedly not make sense, and if you don't challenge it, they'll make you pay it.

Here are a couple of tips:

1.  Communicate, and communicate nicely. The old saying, "You get more with honey than with vinegar" holds true when you're speaking to professionals that are used to being yelled at. Can you imagine? I have so much respect for someone who goes to work to answer phones of angry patients that have "medical bill shock." That's such a thankless job. They did not make your bill high or wrong, yet people take their frustrations out on them. If you're nice, respectful, but to the point and direct, you'll get the answers and/or direction that you need.

2.  If you have an outpatient, non-emergent test, imaging study, or laboratory exam, call around. Shop for the best the price. Where the hospital or insurance company tells you to go may not be what's best for you, or your wallet. A simple Google search will bring up a plethora of outpatient imaging centers and laboratories, including labs that don't require a provider's order. Call them and ask for your insurance price and a cash price for a service. You can't really do that in the ER, so you are pretty much at the mercy of the hospital at that point.

3.  After you receive your hospital bill, negotiate the price. Ask for a payment plan, and offer to pay what you feel you can afford. The key here is to not just ignore the bills. They won't magically go away, and they'll report you to a collection agency if you fall behind without a plan in place. I once paid $0.05 on a medical bill, just to keep the payment period active and in good standing. These hospitals can't call you delinquent if you're making payments on your bill.

Worker's compensation is an entirely different type of insurance, and I don't find many people talking about it. It's really important to know and understand your rights if you get hurt at work. I feel the main reason for this is that your private health insurance does not cover work-related injuries.

Imagine this. You roll your ankle while moving a few heavy plants at the local hardware store. You swear and dance and "walk it off," but two days later, the pain is still there, or maybe it's worse. You decide to go in to your local urgent care to get the injured area examined. You don't tell them it happened at work, or they didn't ask you. An x-ray is taken, and it looks like you actually broke the tip of your fibula, i.e., the smaller, long leg bone on the outside of your leg. You were still able to walk, but you need to see an orthopedist to get it repaired.

When you see the orthopedist, you tell them about the injury in more detail. Their office will confirm that it's work related and schedule you for surgery.

When your private insurance sees that note, they can deny all claims related to that incident. So you'll get 100% price bills for the previous visits, and if you needed surgery, you'd have to pay cash for that.

You then call and inform your boss. You didn't initially file an accident report, so they're reluctant to say it truly happened at work. Even if they do complete the paperwork, their worker's compensation insurance will certainly have questions as to why it wasn't filed in the beginning.

You see the mess this can cause? I've seen people also charged with insurance fraud because they knowingly filed a work-related injury under private insurance. No good.

Companies and businesses are required to carry such insurance. If you get hurt at work, make sure you use it. Even if worker's compensation picks up the claim after you tried to file under your private insurance, why give yourself the headache?

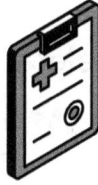

# CHAPTER 7
## BASIC ANATOMY

*If you don't know anatomy, you don't know shit!*

–Joshua Yellen

The key to understanding the human body begins with understanding the parts of the human body. Remember back in kindergarten? "The thigh bone is connected to the... knee bone!" We get a basic grasp of who we are and how we're designed in grammar school, but then the information fades unless you go to school to learn it. This chapter will attempt to give you a better understanding of anatomical terms and conditions, but will fall incredibly short of giving you a comprehensive understanding of all the inner workings of a human being. My goal is to get you to interact with your provider and understand more of what they tell you with regard to a specific condition. If I could get you to provide a report to a paramedic, and they nod their head in amazement and understanding, I'll feel like I won the lottery.

There are 206 bones in the human body, about 600 muscles, 78 organs in 11 organ systems and approximately 37 trillion living cells.

# The Skeletal System

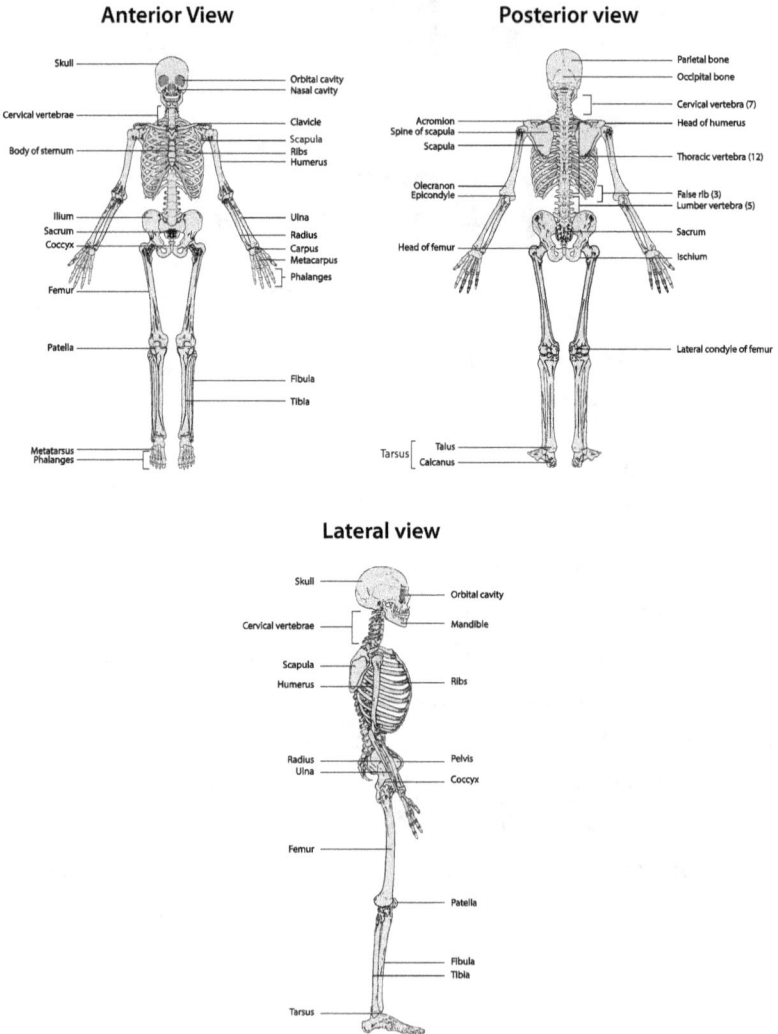

## Anterior View

Skull
Orbital cavity
Nasal cavity
Cervical vertebrae
Clavicle
Scapula
Body of sternum
Ribs
Humerus
Ilium
Ulna
Sacrum
Radius
Coccyx
Carpus
Metacarpus
Phalanges
Femur
Patella
Fibula
Tibia
Metatarsus
Phalanges

## Posterior view

Parietal bone
Occipital bone
Cervical vertebra (7)
Acromion
Head of humerus
Spine of scapula
Scapula
Thoracic vertebra (12)
Olecranon
False rib (3)
Epicondyle
Lumber vertebra (5)
Sacrum
Head of femur
Ischium
Lateral condyle of femur
Tarsus
Talus
Calcanus

## Lateral view

Skull
Orbital cavity
Cervical vertebrae
Mandible
Scapula
Humerus
Ribs
Radius
Pelvis
Ulna
Coccyx
Femur
Patella
Fibula
Tibia
Tarsus

68

All of these cells must work in harmony, or chaos ensues. This might seem overwhelming, and frankly, it can be. It's often a challenge to keep it all straight, and it's easy to be confused. Like my PA school mentor told me, "You eat an elephant one bite at a time." I'm going to break down the body's 11 organ systems into one chapter in an easy-to-read book. Let's discuss a few body systems.

The first is the circulatory system. This includes structures like your heart, your blood vessels, such as arteries, veins and capillaries, and the blood itself. Think of this system like a big plumbing circuit, a circuit that's actually miles long. The role of the circulatory system is to circulate your blood to all areas of your body. Your blood contains oxygen that is carried away from the heart and to the rest of the body in the arteries, and your veins carry used, deoxygenated blood back to the heart, and eventually the lungs to deliver and excrete carbon dioxide, the waste product that we produce after using oxygen.

In keeping with the plumbing analogy, if these components are under too much pressure, as in the case with hypertension, or high blood pressure, pipes (i.e., veins and arteries) can burst. High blood pressure can cause all sorts of problems; trouble with your eyes, kidneys, heart, and brain. If the pressure is too low, all the nutrients in your blood won't be adequately accessible to your body. This is why you lose consciousness if you don't have enough blood getting to your brain.

Your heart is a four-chamber pump that regulates and controls the flow of the pipes. It's a complex structure that is positioned in the center of your chest, and it's not heart- shaped like your Hallmark cards would suggest. It's more like the size and shape of your fist, if you hold your fist over your breastplate, or sternum.

Your heart essentially runs off a series of electrical shocks that cause a contraction in a specific part of the heart. These shocks work in the background without you having to think about it. A series of chemical reactions causes these shocks—and therefore your heart muscles--to contract in just the right way. When you feel your heartbeat, i.e., your pulse, on your wrist or neck, you're feeling the wave of blood pushed by that muscle contraction in your heart.

Your heart has its own pipes that supply blood to the heart muscle. When people have a heart attack, those pipes get clogged to the point where not enough blood could supply the muscle, and the muscle basically suffocates.

Your blood is composed of several ingredients. Hemoglobin is the little red donut that transports the oxygen in the blood. If you don't have enough hemoglobin in your blood, you can't transport enough oxygen. This is called anemia. If the donuts aren't shaped correctly, you could have a disease called sickle cell anemia.

The respiratory system deals with air, specifically getting it from the outside to the inside of your body, and regulating the body's pH balance. This includes your lungs, trachea, and respiratory airways. As we breathe, air travels into the aveoli of the lungs where the transfer of oxygen and carbon dioxide occur. These aveoli look like balloons or clusters of grapes, and they act like a train station of sorts. Oxygen boards the train, aka the capillaries, and carbon dioxide exits the train. The lungs also help us regulate our pH balance by removing the right amount of carbon dioxide, which is an acid. Unfortunately acid/base regulation is entirely too complex for this book.

One common condition that affects the respiratory system is Chronic Obstructive Pulmonary Disease, or COPD. This often occurs in smokers, where the aveoli get damaged to the point where they can't appropriately transfer oxygen and carbon dioxide. Asthmatics have situations where their airways narrow and/or fill with mucus. This makes it difficult to move air, and the narrowing of the airways create a whistling sound that we call wheezing.

If air gets outside the chest cavity, it's usually caused by a spontaneous or traumatic pneumothorax. This is serious, because the air will impede the lungs from expanding and contracting. The more you try to breathe, the more air seeps into the chest cavity. This is treated by "decompressing" the chest, usually with a needle.

The lymphatic system is the body's trash compactor. I often suggest visualizing a medieval battle as an example of what the lymphatic system does. When the battle concludes, the townspeople clear the battlefield of all the "remnants." Your lymphatic system is the body's transport system for elements that are not blood. Think bacteria, extra fluid, fats, and other substances. The parts of the lymphatic system are the lymph nodes, lymph ducts, vessels, and glands. This system also transports antibodies and white blood cells, which are our fighter cells that fend off viruses and bacteria.

Lymph nodes can get clogged and subsequently infected. In addition, lymph nodes play a role in staging cancer. If cancer cells enter the lymphatic system, those cells can then spread rapidly to other systems of the body.

The largest body system is the integumentary system, which is your skin. Most people don't think of their skin as an organ or a body system, but consider how important your skin is. Your skin is responsible for keeping dangerous elements away from your internal organs, fighting off infection, and keeping us cool via sweating. Your peripheral nerves are considered part of this system as well. So all of your sensations of pressure, pain, and temperature come from the numerous peripheral nerves in this system.

The endocrine system is an incredibly complex network of organs that regulate the body's hormone production. This includes organs such as the thyroid, pituitary gland, thymus, pineal gland, adrenal glands, pancreas, ovaries, and testes. Hormones are messenger cells that give specific instructions to certain cells or organs. Too much or too little of any hormone will cause issues. Diabetes is a common hormonal disorder that is triggered by the pancreas' inability to produce enough insulin. This causes your blood sugar to increase. Women can suffer from Polycystic Ovarian Syndrome, or PCOS, which will affect female estrogen levels. Hyperthyroidism and hypothyroidism occur when your thyroid produces too much or too little hormones.

The nervous system is equally complex, and the medical community continues to learn and discover more and more about the workings of your brain and spinal cord. Your brain is your computer. It takes all the information received from your central and peripheral nervous system and processes it. Some of this is voluntary, like moving your arms or reading this book, and some of it is involuntary, like your heart beating. Just think about the processing power it would take for a computer to process just one second of brain power. This was attempted in 2013,[29][30] and it took the world's largest computer at the time, with 83,000 processors, and 40 minutes, to compute what the brain's 100 billion nerve cells do in one second. To put this in perspective, scientists believe the Milky Way galaxy contains about 80- to 100 billion stars. We have that many nerve cells in our head.

Basically, I'm saying the human computer is pretty powerful. It's also incredibly sensitive. It's the only organ system that's not supplied by blood. Rather, cerebrospinal fluid (CSF) bathes these structures. A CSF infection is terribly serious and requires hospital care.

The GI system mentioned in a previous section is also called "the gut" and comprises everything from the mouth to the rectum, and everything in between. This system is responsible for consuming, breaking down, digesting, absorbing, and expelling our food and nutrients. We have learned more in the last several years about how important gut health truly is to our overall health, and more literature continues to emerge that ties gut health to diseases like anxiety and depression, Alzheimer's disease, Parkinson's, as well as dermatologic conditions and autoimmune disorders.

The GI tract can be as long as 30 feet in some individuals, and the time it takes for food to traverse the system is around 50 hours. Digestion begins immediately with the introduction of saliva to the food. Once the food reaches the stomach, food is further broken down by hydrochloric acid and other enzymes. These acids are potent enough to dissolve a nail, so it's best these acids stay where they're supposed to. When acid enters the esophagus, that's when you get Gastroesophageal Reflux Disease, or GERD.

I'll address diet in another chapter, but I can't stress this enough. If you want to keep the doctor away, it's paramount that you're eating a diet that is consistent with healthy living. *So* many diseases can be prevented with proper nutrition.

Of course, there are issues that are often out of your control. One is appendicitis. Your appendix is a little rat tail that is attached at the base of your large intestine. If this structure gets inflamed or infected, it can burst, emptying material inside the sterile abdominal cavity. This is, of course, dangerous, and it's important to recognize appendicitis before that rupture occurs.

So if you're laying on the floor with belly pain that only worsens with time (like I was on Christmas day in 2021), you may want to get that evaluated.

The urinary system consists of the bladder, kidneys, ureter, and urethra. This system is how you excrete toxins and waste from your body. The kidneys filter your blood and help remove excess fluid from your body, which in turn, regulates your blood pressure.

Kidney function is crucial to overall health and well-being. A poorly functioning kidney can mean an increased buildup of toxins in our system. Urinary Tract Infections (UTIs) are incredibly common—more in females than males—and can sometimes be treated without the need of western medicine. Sometimes.

The musculoskeletal system (my personal favorite) is composed of all our bones, and the ligaments, tendons, and skeletal muscles that are attached to them. Our bones and muscles give us our "frame" and the ability to move the way we do. Our unique structure allows us to jump, dance, sprint, sit, grasp, and walk upright.

The musculoskeletal system is my favorite because it's simple to understand. Human biomechanics makes sense to me. From a medical standpoint, it's either broken, or it's not. It's torn, or it's not torn. We either rely on the body to heal itself, or we intervene in the form of surgery. It's very black and white, with very few exceptions. We will talk more about bones and joints in a later chapter.

The reproductive system is the only one that requires another person (or medical intervention) to complete its intended mission. As the name implies, the reproductive system is responsible for reproducing, in the form of tiny humans. As I'm writing this book, this system has come under a bit of scrutiny and controversy, but I assure you, the science is still clear: Males are born with one set of reproductive organs, and females are born with a different set of organs. One requires the other to reproduce.

In my opinion, males have it pretty easy with regard to the reproductive system. Sure, men can have medical issues in the reproductive tract such as testicular cancer, erectile dysfunction and prostatitis, among other things. Females have a laundry list of conditions that need to be monitored and treated if they arise. Females also have a monthly menstrual cycle that requires attention from the time they hit puberty (usually around 12 years old) until they hit menopause around 50. This is why women have gynecologists that specialize in female reproductive disorders.

As far as the particular parts go, there are medical conditions in which the genitalia does not form correctly, or the genitalia is ambiguous. This is caused by hormonal imbalances during pregnancy, and there can be associated genetic mutations and malformations. These individuals sometimes cannot reproduce. Note that this is pretty rare.

Males can have testicular issues, including infection, fluid collection, dilated veins in the scrotum (called varicoceles) and even emergent conditions like testicular torsion, where the testes get twisted, which is very painful.

Females can suffer from a litany of conditions, including cancer, issues with menstruation, and yes, pregnancy is considered a medical condition.

Now, if you thought any of those systems were confusing, the immune system might take the cake. There's not a particular organ that makes up the immune system. Rather, it is comprised of elements and components of other systems. Its function is to keep the other systems safe and healthy. Our white blood cells (WBCs) are the foundation of our immune system. There are several different types of WBCs, all designed to perform different functions. Some seek out foreign pathogens. Others flag those pathogens, and others still destroy the "bad guys."

Our immune system is also responsible for allergic responses that we have to food, medications, or the environment around us. The "immune response" is simply the body attacking a particle that might not necessarily be harmful to us, like pollen or cat hair. This response can be mild and cause watery eyes or a skin rash. Some people have severe responses where they can't breathe. These are called anaphylactic reactions. These are bad, and the patient needs emergent care. This is why some people carry pens that contain the medication epinephrine. This medication can reverse the reaction to allow the patient to breathe again.

You could write complete textbooks on any one system I've listed. In fact, it's already been done hundreds of times. If you take away anything from all this information, understand that there are simple ways to deconstruct most disease processes. Learn and understand the basics, so when you speak to a professional, you'll be able to ask additional (and informed) questions and not be completely confused with what you're hearing.

I've provided some diagrams in the back of the book that will help explain some common medical terms. For example, a "fracture" defines any break in a bone, not just a crack. So when a provider tells you you "fractured" a certain bone, it's still broken. There are terms that further describe that fracture, such as "displaced" or "nondisplaced", comminuted, spiral, oblique, etc.

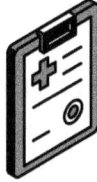

# CHAPTER 8

## BACTERIA VS. VIRUS (VS. ALLERGY)

*It is no measure of health to be well adjusted to a profoundly sick society.*

–Jiddu Krishnamurti

There's not a shift that goes by in an Urgent Care facility or Emergency Room where the difference between viruses and bacterial infections are not explained. Even when I'm not at work, I feel like I have a friend calling me or an acquaintance reaching out on Facebook about "writing them an antibiotic for their sinus infection." I've gone through several responses to this discussion throughout my career. Frankly, it really angers me that providers throw antibiotics at whatever walks into their office. I'm further annoyed at the provider that "gives in" to their patient demand/request and just gives the patient what they want in order to keep their patient satisfaction scores up. As I've gotten older, I've realized there are a lot of reasons why we ended up in this position as a society, where the general public believes that antibiotics are the answer to all of their health problem(s).

I see this especially often in urgent care and family practice offices. I hope to bring some clarification to this today.

So, what is a virus?

**Vi·rus** /ˈvīrəs/ *n. An infective agent that typically consists of a nucleic acid molecule in a protein coat, is too small to be seen by light microscopy, and is able to multiply only within the living cells of a host.*

If we return to middle school biology for a second, a virus is a tiny creature with one purpose—replication. There are hundreds of thousands of viruses that affect humans, and there are millions more that affect plants, animals, bacteria, etc. Viruses have been around much longer than humans, and like cockroaches, they'll probably outlive us, too.

Even if you feel completely healthy, your body is harboring numerous viruses at any given time. It's just part of human life. They need a host to survive, and while some viruses can live on inert surfaces for varying amounts of time, they would eventually die off if they don't have a host in which to reside and thrive.

So Arden, how come are we able to survive and maintain our health if we're constantly inundated with viruses? Humans are blessed with the immune system, and this immune system is able to (under most circumstances) sufficiently prevent viral replication throughout our lives. Even when you're sick, odds are that your immune system will prevent viruses from destroying you.

That said, people still die from viruses. More specifically, they die from complications from the viral illness. Most who die from a viral attack are on the younger or older end of the lifecycle. The younger ones have a less mature immune system that is not completely developed, while the older population has several factors stacked against them, including immune system deficiency, reduced kidney function, and a decrease in overall activity. They also may live in a setting that introduces them to more viruses, such as a group home or retirement center.

So do you need to "treat" viruses? Do you need to rush to your local provider and seek medical care for your cold? As with most things in medicine, and in the voice of my PA school professor, "It depends."

As I promised earlier, here are some ways to effectively self-treat many illnesses or conditions.

If you have a "cold," also known as a viral illness, an upper respiratory illness/infection, the sniffles, etc., the treatment goal is to keep yourself (or the patient), comfortable. If you do nothing at all, the virus is most likely to run its course, and your body's immune system will overcome the offending pathogen. That said, we have made amazing strides in "comfort medicine." There are "western" treatments, e.g., cold and flu medicine, nasal sprays, and 90% of what's on your local pharmacy's "cold and flu" shelves. In addition, there are plenty of homeopathic remedies as well, such as lemon tea and honey, elderberry, vitamin supplements, and many more. I'm a fan of pretty much all of these.

One option I particularly like is nasal sinus rinsing. I hope to complement this book with my own sinus rinse device. I recommend it so much, I should at least make a profit off it. Many people are familiar with neti pots, but I personally don't recommend them. If used incorrectly, they can be very dangerous. Alternatively, I like the sinus bulbs, which are pint-sized bottles that contain a salt water/saline mixture that you squeeze into your nose. If you can tolerate the somewhat weird feeling of having salt water surge up into your nose, that rush will mechanically irrigate congested nasal passages and provide some significant relief. And since it's not medicated, you can use it multiple times per day. Water is the best expectorant on Earth. There is no better medication.

If I'm prescribing medication for a cold, I follow this same thought process. My goal is to reduce your symptoms. I consider prescription cough medicine, nasal sprays, steroids, and other medications to help the particular patient with their specific symptoms.

Let's continue.

**Bac·te·ri·um** /ˌbakˈtirēəm/ *n. 1. bacteria (plural noun). A member of a large group of unicellular microorganisms which have cell walls but lack organelles and an organized nucleus, including some that can cause disease.*

Bacterial infections are apparently what everyone worries about. It's the most common "complaint" I hear from patients when they refer to their sinuses or their cough. Luckily, this is not what humans suffer from most of the time when referring to those symptoms. We'll get into that in a second.

One big difference between viruses and bacteria involves how they survive. Bacteria do not necessarily need a host to keep them alive. Have you ever noticed that reddish-orange ring or film you get in the toilet or shower in your bathroom? That's commonly a family of bacteria called *Klebsiella*. Bacteria can live on inert surfaces, like door handles, chairs, your skin... pretty much anywhere. They can flourish there, in fact. For example, many of us have heard—or personally experienced—the joy of having a "staph infection." This bug is known as *Staphylococcus aureus (S. Aureus)*, or staph, and it's probably living on your skin right now. Two-thirds of all humans on Earth are carriers of staph. It likes to live under the fingernails and in your nose, which is why healthcare workers should always keep their nails clean and trimmed.

I believe staph gets a bad rap. Sure, it kills people. It can be quite devastating; it causes deep skin infections, called cellulitis, abscesses, pneumonia, all sorts of conditions. But like I just mentioned, staph is literally everywhere. Have you ever gotten a little pimple on your face or legs after shaving? Sure you have. Guess what? That was probably a "staph infection." Called folliculitis, these little zits are more common than you can imagine, yet they resolve themselves on their own, or with very mild medical intervention. If we're looking at statistics of all contracted "infections" from the bug, dying from a staph infection is incredibly rare. Is it something we need to pay attention to? Treat when it gets out of control? Absolutely. After all, that's one of the advantages of modern medicine: We have the ability to literally save your life when you'd otherwise die, or be in very poor condition, if not for the advancements we've made in the last 100 years.

Now, back to bacteria.

There are several ways humans can contract bacteria that results in infections. We mentioned *S. Aureus*, which is an opportunistic skin bug. It will make its way into tiny cuts, abrasions, hair follicles, or open wounds. It loves freshly shaven skin since we're opening those pores and exposing them. It's like a highway for bacteria. This is why a good quality skincare regimen is important. I won't sell you on products here; just understand it's a good idea to cleanse the skin after shaving.

Other ways to contract a bacterial infection include inhaling tainted air, and ingesting it when we eat. In females especially, bacteria can enter via your urinary tract. Your immune system still plays a huge role here. Remember: Your immune system is constantly at war with the outside world. We humans are the species we are today, in large part, because of our heavily evolved immune system. So once a bacterial infection takes hold of us (e.g., a bad cellulitis, abscess, pneumonia, UTI, etc.), it'll usually continue to progress and worsen unless medicine is introduced. In other words, that cellulitis will continue to spread, that pneumonia will worsen, and that UTI will progress to the next structure, i.e., the kidneys. That bacteria, like humans, have an innate will to live, and left untreated, they'll continue to spread until they kill the host.

A famous case of fatal bacterial infections include the Legionnaires' disease outbreak in 1976. Attendees of the American Legion convention in Philadelphia were exposed to the deadly Legionella bacteria that had been festering in the air conditioning system at the now closed Bellevue-Stratford Hotel. This airborne bacteria infected guests from age 39 to 82, and 29 people eventually passed away from the illness.

People begin to get really sick when these infections spread. Fulminant pneumonia is a nasty infection that can often require inpatient hospital care. If the bacteria get into our heavily guarded bloodstream, it leads to sepsis. The bloodstream is the highway system for the body, and just like the "good guys" can use the highway, the "bad guys" can use it also. Bacteria in the blood stream have free reign to enter other areas of the body.

Put bluntly, bacterial infections, if left to their own devices, will kill the host unless there is some sort of intervention. This is one issue that modern medicine has achieved that we all need to celebrate–antibiotics.

Antibiotics aren't necessarily new. Civilizations used plants and even moldy bread to treat infections as far back as ancient Egypt. Bacterial infections were the number one human killer in the developed world until the early 20th century when penicillin was "accidentally" discovered by Alexander Fleming.[31] Since the mass production of penicillin, we have learned so much about antibiotics, bacteria, and how bacteria "learns" and adjusts to our treatments.

This leads me to my single biggest issue about the ways medical professionals treat their patients.

**Antibiotics only treat bacterial infections. Antibiotics do not work on viruses.**

This is a pretty straightforward statement. We're taught this in school, and it's embedded in our brains: Too many providers write antibiotics for viruses.

It's become so commonplace that patients come into clinics asking for antibiotics by name.

Before I say another word, read this: If your provider wants to prescribe an antibiotic for you, and you don't know why, ask. It's *your* body, and the consequences are yours if there's an adverse reaction.

There are a couple of problems with inappropriately taking antibiotics. First, any time you put something in your body, your body responds to it. Be it food, drugs, anything. Your body is programmed to break that substance down and use it as fuel. With drugs, every drug ever created has potential side effects. This doesn't mean that you *will* have side effects, but it can happen. Some of these side effects can be minor, like like nausea and upset stomach. Others can be severe, and result in life-changing side effects. From delirium, neuropathy, tumors, and suicidal ideations, to severe secondary yeast infections, a gastrointestinal bacterial subinfection called *C. Difficile,* which causes terrible diarrhea and can ultimately kill you, and Stevens Johnson Syndrome, where your skin literally blisters and sloughs off. Antibiotics are not without risks.

In addition to the side effects, there is a public health concern with people taking antibiotics inappropriately. As we providers continue to prescribe antibiotics when they're not needed, we see an increase in bacterial resistance in these bugs that are repeatedly exposed to the same antibiotic. One metaphor involves walking into your office every day, only to be greeted with a slap in the face when you opened your office door. You may be tricked once or twice, but soon, you're going to find a way to avoid that big whack to your face every day. These bugs are no different. They can be smart, and after many generations of bacterial lifespans, they grow tolerant of the typical drugs we throw at them. That makes something that was typically easy to treat—an ear infection or UTI—a living nightmare for that patient.

Recently, at the time of writing this book, medical guidelines were changed with regard to treating a common sexually transmitted disease (STD). We used to treat the common STD chlamydia with the antibiotic azythromycin. Now, due to bacterial resistance, we had to switch to a stronger medication, called doxycycline. I personally hope this doesn't get worse.

So in case you didn't process what I'm saying, apply these "rules" to your program. If you're prescribed an antibiotic, know and understand why. When you're satisfied with the reason/s, ensure you take it correctly. Also, even though you'll likely feel better two days after starting that antibiotic, finish it. Take all of it. Don't leave any leftover for a rainy day. Bad idea, don't do it.

I want to talk about fever, because it is an issue that patients are always concerned about, and it usually is included in the virus vs. bacteria conversation. And I'll start with saying this:

**I don't really care what your temperature is.**

First, "fever" is technically a measured temperature greater than 100.4 F. Your "fever" at home of 99.8 F is not impressive and doesn't help me at all. I'm sorry you feel bad, but knowing your subclinical temperature won't help the medical community solve the problem.

Fever is the body's natural response to injury or illness. There are studies that prove fever is beneficial to one's recovery. There's is a point of diminishing returns, and even a point where a severely high temperature can be detrimental, e.g., organ damage and death. But this is a high temperature, say 106 F. When you feel bad and have a temperature of 101 or 102 F, I don't really care. All it tells me is that you're sick. It's a nonspecific finding and only part of the entire clinical picture.

I may see a patient with a temperature that raises a suspicion that I am dealing with a possible medical problem like pneumonia or an ear infection, for example. But that's not always the case. You can just have a cold, or viral upper respiratory illness, and have a fever. Long story short, fever can be your friend. Kids with febrile illnesses who remain untreated have been shown to heal faster than if you were to treat them with fever-reducing medications.

There are several ways to accurately measure your temperature. Whichever way choose, ensure you have the right equipment. Don't try to take your temperature under your tongue with one of those infrared scanners. That's not going to work. The container that holds your thermometer will tell you where it's calibrated to measure. Follow the instructions included with the method you select for the job.

Let's bust a myth. If you're sick, and you don't have a fever, you're still contagious. Contagiousness is measured by symptoms, not fever.

Fever is convenient for daycare centers and grammar schools because it's an objective measurement. While I will agree that if you have a clinical fever (>100.4 F), you're likely sick; the absence of fever doesn't make you "healthy." I tell my patients that when it comes to fever, if that's your only symptom, feel free to be around other people and go to work/school. If you're without a clinical fever, but you're coughing around other people, go ahead and stay home. But if you have a clinical fever, I'll bet you likely have at least a symptom or two. Not always, but I'd put a dollar or two on that bet.

So let's talk about fever reducing medications for a second. Acetaminophen (Tylenol®) and ibuprofen (Motrin®, Advil®, etc.) are most commonly used to break a fever and make us feel better. But how do you actually take it? Just because these medications can be found at every pharmacy, store, gas station, or retail place in the world doesn't mean that they can't hurt you. In fact, taking too much of either of these drugs can kill you. An overdose on acetaminophen is not pretty. It shuts down your liver and kills your organs. Overdosing on ibuprofen (a Non-Steroidal Anti-Inflammatory Drug, or NSAIDS) can literally burn a hole in your stomach.

I typically remind patients is how much you can take in a day and how often you can take it. For fever-reducing meds like Tylenol®, the maximum dose in a day is 4,000 milligrams. That means you can take 1,000 milligrams every six hours. With regard to NSAIDS, you can take 2,400 milligrams in a day, or 600 milligrams every six hours.

For an added benefit, alternate the two medications every three hours. The medications have good synergy and work well together.

Remember what I said earlier: All medications have side effects and contraindications. These classes of drugs are no different. If you have liver problems, stay away from Tylenol®. If you have stomach or kidney problems, keep clear of NSAIDS. And of course, talk to your doctor if you have any concerns.

Let's say you're in pain, and it's bad enough to go to the hospital. The hospital staff is going to reach for these medications first, unless there's an obvious reason to look for something stronger, e.g., a broken bone. So if you're headed to the ER for pain, don't be shocked when they hand you something OTC. They're also going to charge you 10 times what the price would be at your local pharmacy.[32]

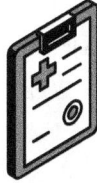

# CHAPTER 9

## HEALTHY LIFESTYLE

*The art of healing comes from nature, not from the physician. Therefore the physician must start from nature, with an open mind.*

—Paracelsus

Oh boy, this is going to be a fun one.

Let me begin by saying this: If you're going to your medical provider for diet help, you're likely not getting the best information. In PA school, I spent maybe one- to two hours on diet and lifestyle changes. Of course, we talked about "making diet and lifestyle changes" when we talked about disease processes. But we never broke down what those changes should actually look like. According to one study, only 15% of physicians were totally comfortable discussing diet with their patients. Even if they were "comfortable" talking about it, what would they actually talk about? You and I can sit here and probably list 25 fad diets from this year alone. There's a new featured diet on the cover of magazines every month.

I'm going to help shed some light on this ever increasingly confusing topic. I'm also going to suggest you do some follow up research here. This topic is complex. Like James Cameron searching for the *Titanic* complex. I'm going to try to keep it light and simple. For bonus reading, I recommend Dr. Paul Saladino's "*The Carnivore Code*" and Dr. Shawn Baker's "*The Carnivore Diet.*"

My approach to diet and healthy living is simple: Eat well, move more. It really is that simple.

Simple does not make it easy, however.

For example, everywhere you turn, you are inundated with pressure, marketing, advertising and "science" that tells you to eat grains, seed oils, processed sugars, and ingredients you can't pronounce. The American Academy of Pediatrics (AAP) recommends children eat fortified cereal, such as Fruit Loops or Cinnamon Toast Crunch. The fact that the AAP has to published an article about limiting rice cereal because it may have too much arsenic[33] in it should tell you all you need to know about how "healthy" these products really are.

I recommended those two "carnivore" books not to persuade you to eat nothing but meat, but to challenge the typical way of thinking. What if I suggested to you that it's the grains and seed oils and processed sugar that's making everyone sick? When I say "sick," I am referring to conditions such as hypertension, dislipidemia (an imbalance of lipids related to cholesterol), and diabetes, all conditions that the typical western medical community will treat you with using medications.

Medications that cause side effects. Side effects that are treated with more medications.

Get the drift?

The fact is, inflammation is the root cause of most—if not all—preventable medical conditions. We are seeing an increase in obesity, cardiovascular events, strokes, diabetes, etc. almost in parallel with the increase of "not real" food in our diets.

Eat real. Eat clean. Move more.

My advice is start by shopping around the perimeter of your grocery store. Start reading ingredient lists. If there's an ingredient that you can't pronounce, or if there's an oil or preservative in the product, put it back on the shelf. I'm a big fan of eating "strict" for a few weeks/months to break the chain that modern western foods have on you. You're addicted to those foods if they're in your diet.[34]

Personally, I'm finding more research favorably supporting the keto and carnivore style of eating than anything on the other end of that spectrum. But whatever you ultimately decide to do, I cannot stress enough how important it is to remove dietary components that create inflammation. This refers to the seed oils and processed foods that sneak into our diet everywhere we turn.

In addition, if you're looking for diet coaching or extra help in this area, be sure to research the nutritional position of your chosen coach/ dietician. You want to establish that their philosophy is in line with yours, after you have sufficiently researched for yourself, of course. This is not the time to find the newest Instagram fad diet coach.

This is one of those situations where you need to start sooner rather than later. While looking at yourself in the mirror and knowing that you have 30-, 40-, 50-plus pounds to lose is intimidating, each weight loss journey starts with a single decision. A single step. Structure your goals as such.

- It's a win if you put your shoes on to go for a walk.
- It's a win if you decide to clean out your pantry.
- It's a win if you chose sugar-free yogurt instead of ice cream.
- Let those wins accumulate, and watch the transformation take place.

Simple, not easy.

Another component that I find to be super helpful (and so do my patients in my current practice), is a mood or gratitude journal. There's a type of journal for just about everything. There are spiritual journals, headache journals, gratitude and mental health journals, even journals to track your menstrual cycle. These journals will provide an incredible resource for your own personal journey, as well as useful information for your treating provider. Just like you forget 90% of what your provider tells you during an office visit, you'll also forget 90% of all the things you feel and experience during a given day. Information is powerful, and it could be the difference between a correct diagnosis and treatment plan and the runaround one gets when the answer isn't clear.

Journaling is also incredible for stress management and clearing your thoughts. A stressed mind is a stressed body, and when you have stress, your immune system becomes compromised. You ever notice that kids spread illness the first week of school, and they also get sick during exam week? I totally understand that kids will do *anything* and *everything* to get out of school. I practically wrote the book on this in my younger years, and there is some validity to this phenomenon.

While its true that kids are being exposed to an influx of shared germs once school begins, stress can play a role in this, too. Stress takes a toll on the body's defense mechanisms, and if you can't defend the influx of viruses and bugs, you get sick.

How's that diet looking?

I ask this question to nearly every patient I encounter. I typically get the same answer: "It's pretty good". "I watch what I eat". "I eat a lot of chicken and salads". Patients that are underweight and morbidly overweight tell me the same things.

I think a more relevant question would be something like this: What are you eating to promote good immune function?

There are plenty of resources and studies[35] that demonstrate which types of foods help boost that immune system. But if I were to break it down for you, here's a few things that might look familiar:

- Wild-caught salmon, and other high Omega-3 fat fish
- High Vitamin C foods like oranges and grapefruit
- Garlic
- Ginger
- Turmeric
- Yogurt
- Honey

Isn't it crazy that Fruit Loops didn't make this list?

I want to touch on one more subject in this chapter that could arguably be a chapter (or book) on its own–supplements.

Full disclosure; I'm a believer in supplements when they meet two criteria:

- The body can't naturally produce what you're giving it.
- There isn't an easy way to get said ingredient/supplement naturally/holistically in your diet.

With these two criteria, most supplements fall short in my opinion. In fact, since there are little to no regulatory restrictions on supplements, I'd go so far to say that most supplements are total garbage. They're likely unnecessary for consumption, as long as you're eating a satisfactory diet that meets your nutritional requirements.

I've seen supplement companies being operated out of garages and warehouses formerly used for car battery storage. In today's world, anyone can start a supplement store. Don't misunderstand me, I'm all for the American dream, and if you want to make it in the supplement industry, certainly go for it. And if it were me, I'd be operating as a supplement developer with the same integrity that I operate my medical practice.

Some people don't. And the truth is that you never fully know what you're getting in these supplements.

One of my favorite supplement "tricks" is the term "proprietary blend." Ever read that on your multivitamin label? It gives these companies the opportunity to put whatever they want into their supplement in order to call it "theirs." Personally, that doesn't give me a confident feeling. If your product is so special, then file for patents and make it legit. Then you can safely let everyone know what you're selling, and you can sue whomever copies it.

And in case you didn't know, supplements—even "good" ones—can interfere with prescription medication. The American Academy of Family Physicians (AAFP) has a decent list of commonly used supplements that can interfere with your meds.[36] While this list isn't exhaustive, I recommend you take this into consideration when considering a new supplement. It's always best to have a relationship with a qualified provider (who will give you more than six minutes of their time) to ask their opinion if you need added assurance. Don't take this section, or this book for that matter, as personal medical advice.

If you absolutely must use a supplement for whatever reason, be it that you don't have access to a quality food source, or simply refuse to eat it for whatever reason, I'm not judging you. Please do your research on the company that's making it. There are reputable companies out there, but they are the exception and not the rule.

All that said, here are some supplements I would recommend:

- vitamins C, D, zinc, quercetin, colloidal silver, magnesium
- protein, creatine, branched-chain amino acids (BCAAs)
- Consider organ meat supplements if you choose not to eat them

Note that some of "grandma's old remedies" should also be considered. Recently, I've been noticing an oldie but goodie floating around social media. Our grandparents would chop onions, put them in a mason jar with garlic cloves, then cover them all in raw, local honey.

It's supposed to be a natural immune booster. Some people swear by it. Consider them on a case-by-case basis.

If you read this far, this shouldn't surprise you. But keep in mind that these miracle supplements that are sold on social media and on overnight infomercials are more likely to become expensive paperweights than offer any real benefit.

I'm not perfect, I've fallen for them too. And they're still in my bathroom cabinet, reminding me of the foolish ways I used to spend money.

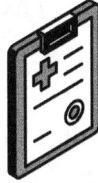

# CHAPTER 10
## SOME TIPS ON BONES

*We are all fixing what is broken. It is the task of a lifetime. We'll leave much unfinished for the next generation.*

–Author Abraham Verghese

I'd be lying if I didn't say orthopedics is a topic close to my heart. I apologize to all my medical aesthetics patients; I love you all. But orthopedics has always just made sense to me. If it's broken, you fix it. If it's torn, either your body or your surgeon repairs it. It's black and white. There's no gray area. Well, there is *a little* of that; after all, it's medicine, and nothing is ever absolute.

I am a prime example of this phenomenon. As I write this, I became the victim of a partially torn anterior cruciate ligament (ACL) in my right knee. It was me vs. a flight of stairs, and the stairs won. I knew immediately that something was going on down there, but it was, understandably, hard for me to evaluate my own knee.

So I put all the practical knowledge I've accumulated thus far, and as I sought care, I got multiple opinions as to what was going on and what

I should do about it. One exam was downright laughable. My urgent care provider did not know how to perform a basic knee exam; I had to teach her. The first surgical opinion I received was aggressive, and to be honest, I was okay with it. My thought was to get it repaired and get the rehabilitation process started. The sooner, the better.

When I got my second surgical opinion, the surgeon who examined me made sense. He evaluated the plain and advanced imaging, and he gave me options. *He gave me options.* This was pretty cool, and his approach impressed me.

So I still may need surgery, but I'm confident in the plan that was offered. Maybe I'll share my outcome in my second book.

The human body has 206 bones and about 600 muscles. Collectively, they create the most complex living, breathing, anatomical structure the universe has ever seen. These muscles and bones work in harmony to create movement. They allow you to walk upright, run, jump, change direction, and twist and turn our frames with ease, depending on who is doing the twisting. These muscles also aid in breathing, which is kind of a big deal. When this harmony is disrupted, injury is imminent.

This can be a slow process, as in the case of tendonitis or stress fractures. This process can be super fast also, like we see in high-impact trauma.

While the treatment of some orthopedic injuries become obvious, such as a leg facing the wrong way, or a dislocation of some sort, some may not be immediately apparent. The goal of this chapter is not to make you an expert in bones and joints, but rather to provide you with some useful and reliable information to help you know when to seek care, where to go, and what to expect.

Let's clarify a few points:

- Fractures and breaks are the same thing. Think of "fracture" as the medical word for "break." Whether it's a tiny crack or it's snapped in half, it's a fracture.

- For the overwhelming majority of cases, ligaments connect bone to bone. Tendons connect muscles to bone.
- You know when you're eating chicken off the bone, and there's that smooth white stuff on the end of the bone? That's cartilage. It covers all our articulating surfaces. We'll talk about that in a bit.
- The body will adapt to the forces that are placed on it (see "Wolff's Law").
- Like a paperclip, ligaments can only take so much force until they become permanently deformed (see "stress/strain principle").
- Every injury, regardless of its size, will produce swelling. How we control and manipulate that swelling will determine how quickly we recover.

The following information contains a significant amount of overlap with previous chapters, which illustrates the importance of "the fundamentals" in practical medical assessment. If you just suffered some sort of bone and joint injury, and you are looking for what to do and where to go, refer back to Chapters 3 and 4.

Let's first talk about what happens, and when, immediately after an injury. [37,38] There are four main stages the experiences, from the moment an injury occurs until you are considered "healed": hemostasis, inflammation, proliferation, and remodeling. When I discuss this phenomenon with my patients, I use the analogy of your local city repairing a pothole in the street.

If your town is anything like my hometown of New Orleans, Louisiana, there are plenty of potholes to reference. If I mention the word "pothole" to my patient, they immediately visualize that abyss of asphalt at their favorite corner or outside their home. We know that, depending on the location of the pothole–and what it's made of–will determine how long it takes for the repair team to get there and repair it.

Once they arrive, they work as fast as they can to put a patch down. We all know that this initial patch isn't the best fix one could achieve. It's usually a bit haphazard and clumsy. Time is considered to be more important than quality work, but one can still drive on it. Eventually, over time, you might get a crew back to the pothole to give it a more thorough repair, but even with the most skilled of workers, it'll never be as it was originally. There will always be indications that something once happened there.

To me, this is the best analogy of what goes on inside (or outside) your body with an injury.

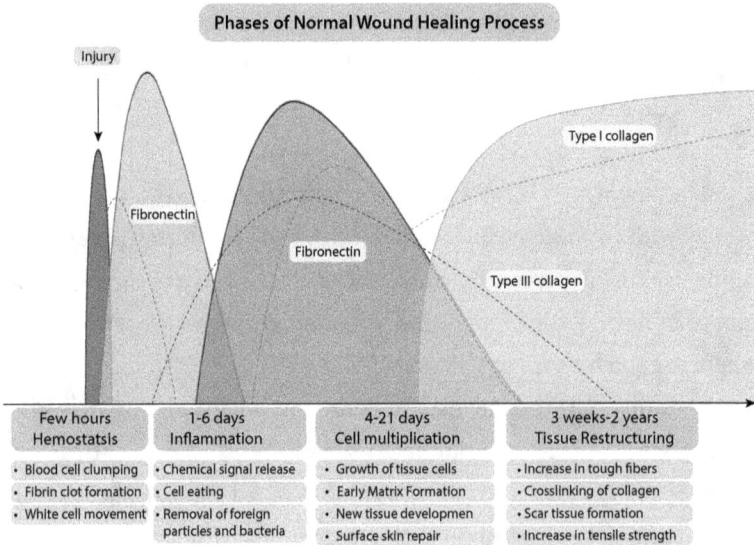

Phases of Normal Wound Healing Process

| Few hours<br>Hemostatsis | 1-6 days<br>Inflammation | 4-21 days<br>Cell multiplication | 3 weeks-2 years<br>Tissue Restructuring |
|---|---|---|---|
| • Blood cell clumping<br>• Fibrin clot formation<br>• White cell movement | • Chemical signal release<br>• Cell eating<br>• Removal of foreign<br>  particles and bacteria | • Growth of tissue cells<br>• Early Matrix Formation<br>• New tissue developmen<br>• Surface skin repair | • Increase in tough fibers<br>• Crosslinking of collagen<br>• Scar tissue formation<br>• Increase in tensile strength |

As I explain the four stages, understand that this pattern for whatever injury that occurs, from your papercut to your massive, high-energy trauma. The repair of the injury varies, but the physiology–the process that occurs behind the scenes–is pretty much the same.

The initial phase is the bleeding phase. Bleeding obviously occurs due to the injury of the vessels involved. If we cut our skin or tear a muscle, those vessels that supply the structure with nutrients will overflow until the clotting phase can occur. Externally, this can last for minutes to hours, depending on what vessels have been disrupted. Internally, this process can last for the first four- to six hours, again, depending on what is damaged.

The next phase, i.e., the inflammatory phase, is often considered to be a negative thing, but inflammation is critically important when considering the healing of the structure. The elements involved in this swelling include helper cells, white blood cells, and other chemical mediators that help remove the dead and damaged tissue and get the body prepared for healing.

Think of inflammation as your body turning on your kitchen faucet. As the faucet is turned on, a rush of liquid flows down to the basin below. It's our job as the person who turned on the faucet to know how much water we need from the faucet, and for how long. With regard to your body, during an injury, your body turns on that faucet rather quickly after an injury, but it doesn't adequately control the amount of the flow. This active swelling phase lasts for one- to three days, and can remain in the area for a few weeks.

The key to a quick recovery from an injury begins with monitoring the amount of swelling that develops at an injury site, and then reducing it in a systematic fashion with rehabilitation and therapeutic modalities such as ice baths, intermittent compression and therapeutic exercise. This process emphasizes the importance of a good athletic trainer, physical therapist, or physiotherapist as part of your team when recovering from an injury.

Proliferation is the "patch job" part of the recovery process. This begins after the acute inflammatory phase, and can last for a month to several weeks after the initial injury. The primary cellular element involved is the fibroblast. Fibroblasts are "builder cells" that assist with developing the supportive netting in our body, connecting different components such as organs and tissues. Fibroblasts ensure a special protein (collagen) keeps this netting strong and in place. This collagen is specified as Type 3 collagen; this is that haphazard repair that I was referring to in my analogy. It's immature and weak; it will not sustain the forces that the body part would normally sustain. The body treats Type 3 collagen like a kid dropping a game of pick-up sticks on the floor; it's random and without true form.

A good therapist understands this process and prescribes exercises and therapeutic modalities to help facilitate this process and align these collagen cells from Type 3 to Type 1, which happens during the next phase of healing.

The remodeling phase is when the tissue starts to become "like new" again. This process commences around three weeks after an injury, and it can last for years. It's time for the body to convert those immature Type 3 collagen fibers into sturdy, organized Type 1 fibers. With the aid of therapy, this process can be accelerated and improved. Therapists will begin stretching and challenging the area with weight-bearing activity and exercises, basically telling the body how to organize those various random fibers. This helps reduce scar tissue and provide it with a chance to heal effectively as it was when you were born. In other words, it gives the pothole the best opportunity to blend in seamlessly with the concrete or asphalt around it.

Understanding this process that's been overly simplified is helpful to understand the "why" behind the healing and rehabilitation process of an injury. If we're talking about a skin injury—such as an abrasion or a laceration—you can apply certain techniques once the area is healed, to help reduce scarring. In addition, with more complex injuries, e.g., an ACL tear or a long bone fracture, once the surgeon repairs the area with a new ligament or some sophisticated hardware, the healing process can begin, and therapy can help accelerate your healing time.

It's important to remember that surgery is basically re-creating an injury. So that particular surgery has its own bleeding, inflammation, remodeling, and proliferation. One real hack is a therapeutic philosophy called prehab, where one starts to rehabilitate an injured area before surgical intervention. This will greatly reduce the healing time on the back end of surgery, and the outcomes are generally more favorable.

Prehab is more prevalent when a fracture is not present because fractures ultimately need to be stabilized before moving them is possible.

We discussed how the remodeling phase can possibly take years, and that's certainly true. But if that's the case, how are people able to return to participating in sports and everyday activities so quickly relative to the healing time? That's because that remodeling phase can assist in determining the strength in the tissue that is "good enough" while still healing. Make no mistake; there are several instances where people return too soon from injury and suffer a re-injury to the affected area. It's a game you have to play, and I highly suggest you have someone familiar with your injuries who can monitor you and give you proper advice. The single best investment you can make in yourself when you're injured is quality physical therapy. Not all physical therapists are created equal. I always recommend a physical therapy group that has experience with active patients recovering from sports medicine-type injuries, even if your injury is not sports related. Why? Because these physical therapists understand what it's like for their athletes to be missing playing time. You'll get better faster, with fewer complications or delays in your recovery.

Okay, enough for the science talk for now. How do you treat these injuries on your own? After all, that's kind of what this book is about.

Let's go back to the moment of the injury. I'm going to use myself and my most recent mishap as a reference. As I'm lying at the bottom of that staircase, uttering some very choice four-letter words, I'm immediately starting to assess my risk. Like I said, I knew *something* was going on in there, but I couldn't really tell how severe it was. My first order of business was to make sure my life wasn't in danger.

Obviously, I'm conscious, breathing, and have a pulse. That's a good thing. What does my knee look like? Is it at least pointing in the right direction? Could an artery or major nerve be damaged? Did I hit my head or neck? Injure my back? Nope, all that is good, I thought. I do some basic palpation of the area and notice I have significant pain on the outside of my knee, close to my fibular head. The fibula is the small, less weight-bearing bone in the lower leg. The pain raises my suspicion because there's a big nerve behind it. Is it broken? As I continue to massage that area, it's sore, but no sharp, intense pain. I don't feel it moving around.

As I'm sitting there, I'm starting to notice the pain subside slightly, and after moving the knee back and forth, I decide it's okay to try to bear some weight. This will provide me with a useful amount information, specifically if I should continue to put weight on it.

And as I stand up, I'm sore, but there's no sharp, stabbing pain, something I would expect if there's a more serious fracture. More good news, I thought to myself.

This all occurred in a matter of 30 seconds, but as I stood there, a bit embarrassed at my middle-aged blunder, I was able to make several decisions based on how I currently felt. Had I had some sort of bleeding issue, crooked appendage, numbness or tingling, or other "bad" symptom, I would have dialed 911 to take myself to the nearest ER. I was able to determine that this issue could be serious (as in I may need surgery on my knee), but at least it wasn't life threatening.

So I just saved myself hours of time and thousands of dollars by *not* seeking emergent care for a nonemergent issue.

When assessing a patient who is injured, there's a simple acronym you must remember to guide you when you're evaluating someone with an injury–BLT–which stands for Bone, Ligament, Tendon. This is more of a secondary assessment, while the ABCs (Airway, Breathing, Circulation) take priority. Personally, the first bones I'm inspecting are the skull and spine, as that can be as serious or life threatening.

If this is you or a loved one, first determine if the life or the limb is at risk. If so, no question, initiate your EAP. If there is no risk of loss of life or limb, you can determine the next course of action.

If I personally witnessed the injury, that gives me a plethora of information, and I can omit several steps involved in assessing the situation. If I did not personally observe what happened, I'll ask a trustworthy and reliable witness. If that's not an option, I begin my questioning with the most serious issue then work my way through to the least serious.

Some of these questions might include:

- What happened?
- Did you hit your head? Does your neck or back hurt?
- Did you lose consciousness?
- What is hurting right now?

If we're assuming the patient suffered a head injury/concussion, I'll pay very close attention to eye movement, breathing rate, and answers to the patient's questions. Concussions alone could be the subject of a book of their own, and they're more serious than any of us thought when I was in school.

At the same time of questioning, I'm making visual assessments and gently palpating areas that may be injured. I'm always checking for head, neck, and spine irregularities first (again, looking for the more serious injury) and working my way around the body, depending on the situation.

It's important to know how to read the room. If I'm walking on a tennis court, and I see a conscious person holding their ankle, I'm probably not going to assess their head and neck very closely; I'm probably going to inspect their ankle. Be thorough, but don't be annoying.

What does a broken bone feel like to the person evaluating an injury? You'll never forget it if you ever feel one. Remember what's happening in there. When you break a bone, the pain comes from the initial trauma, then the pain gets worse when those fractured pieces grinding against each other. So when you palpate a broken bone, the patient does not like it. You'll be able to accurately determine where a fracture is once you palpate it.

If you suspect a fracture (or if it's obvious), don't overly manipulate it. Maintain some decency, as often people in this situation are sensitive to being excessively touched. Your job is to stabilize this fracture and make the appropriate determination on where to go and what to do about it.

When you stabilize a fracture, it's important to understand where the fracture is and what joint(s) are involved. You must stabilize the joint above and below the fracture site. So if the ulna (forearm) is suspected to be broken, you would stabilize both the wrist and the elbow. If it's a suspected fibula fracture in the ankle, you can either use a short posterior leg splint, or you can apply a longer splint and include the knee. When in doubt, splint more.

If you suspect a femur fracture, you're probably calling EMS. If EMS isn't an option, you require something called a femur traction splint to keep the bone in line. This isn't something you pick up at Walmart. You need to know what you're doing when applying one of those. I'll eventually offer a course and a means to purchase one if you're so inclined. Keep an eye on my website for details.

If you don't have a femur traction splint, and EMS isn't close by, you have to improvise. Poles, pool cues, fence posts etc. can be used as a splint in the event of an emergency. Be sure to check for pulses away from the injury site. I always travel with multiple tourniquets for this very reason. If bloodflow is compromised and a vessel is damaged, things can go bad quickly without a tourniquet.

Splinting material could be nearly anything you have at your disposal. Popsicle sticks, twigs/branches, even rolled up newspapers can be used to keep a fracture stable. I always advocate to keep some structural aluminum malleable (SAM) splints handy, but if these aren't available, use whatever you have nearby to reduce your patient's pain and chance for secondary injury. You can create a sturdy splint later; use what you have to keep the patient comfortable and facilitate healing.

I think it's important that if you're reading this book, and are in the position to put this information to use, please be as conservative as possible. I'd rather splint something I think is fractured and be wrong than not splinting, which would result in the injury not properly recovering.

Muscle, tendon, and ligament injuries are likely not going to be life-threatening, but the injury could still be debilitating, and it could take a long time to heal. One-thousand page books have been written to instruct practitioners on how to assess, treat, repair, and rehabilitate these types of injuries, so I don't expect these few pages to make you an expert.

Here are a couple of points to keep in mind if you happen to assess injuries such as these:

- Most patients won't want to move the affected area after an injury such as an ACL tear or rotator cuff injury. There's a phenomenon that occurs called "guarding." You've probably seen this watching your favorite sports team play on TV. When someone gets injured, they tend to position that joint/body part as still and immobile as possible. Arms are placed across the chest and belly, as if they're already in a sling. When one has a knee injury, one can find them laying down, holding the knee, with the knee slightly flexed.

- When you are testing ligaments to see if they're injured, you're essentially pulling or pushing along the ligament's intended vector of protection. For example, your ACL in your knee is designed to keep your tibia in your lower leg from sliding forward. When you tear this ligament, there's nothing really preventing the tibia from slipping, and the patient feels it. It's often described as "unstable," or "my leg feels like a wet noodle." If you understand how ligaments are supposed to work, you can test to determine if they're damaged or intact.

- Muscle injuries are interesting. We grade muscle "strains" in three stages. A Grade 1 strain indicates stretching of muscle fibers. Clinically, this causes pain, swelling, but not a significant amount of dysfunction. They hurt, you hobble around, and they improve in a few weeks. Grade 2 strains involve some muscle fiber tearing. These usually bruise pretty significantly, and in the some patients, you can actually palpate the "divot and ball" deformity. If you can, visualize the muscle fibers tearing and rolling up upon themselves, as if you were scooping ice cream from the top of the tub. Grade 3 strains are tears. Ruptures. Bad. Surgical intervention is often required. The tell-tale sign is that the patient will not be able to use that muscle the way it is intended, and there's usually some sort of visual deformity.

As you can imagine, most of these injuries hurt. Swelling and pain are quite synonymous with acute musculoskeletal injuries, big and small, and it's important to be aware that the medical community overtreats pain. Depending on where you go for treatment after one of these injuries, you could very easily get a bag full of prescriptions for some pretty serious medications for pain like Percocet, Norco®, gabapentin, oxycodone and more.

If you learn one thing from this book, learn this: The medical community began and perpetuated the opioid crisis. You do not need opiates to recover from an injury. Pain, to some extent, is good for you. And as mentioned previously, you *need* some swelling to promote healing. Anti-inflammatories could lead to delayed healing.

Did you know that the active ingredient in opiates like Percocet and Norco® is not the opiate? It's actually acetaminophen, i.e., Tylenol®.

The ingredient that is actually modulating your pain is the Tylenol® that's compounded with the opiate; the latter simply makes you high.

You'd be surprised what level of pain you can actually tolerate when you're injured. I advise you to use that medication as sparingly as possible, and once your pain is gone, return the unused prescription to your pharmacy.

That's right; return your meds. Most pharmacies have either "bring back days" where you can clean out your medicine cabinet, or they will be eager to take those meds off your hands. Keeping them can result in theft, taking the medications by mistake, or having them used for recreational purposes. Flushing it will contaminate the water system, which is a contributing factor as to why our water supply is poisoning us. That's a topic for another book, too.

The last condition I'll discuss with regard to orthopedics is arthritis. Remember me explaining cartilage earlier? I used the chicken bone analogy as your visual. I'll make a bold statement here: Arthritis only happens for two reasons. First, you have overused a joint, or you're too fat. That's it. More people are getting knee and hip replacements now compared to 20 years ago. Has knee/hip/shoulder replacement technology changed that much? Not really, but people are getting fatter.

Imagine this. You're a 200-pound male, walking down the street. Every time your heel hits the ground, you're exerting force onto the pavement, and there is a reactionary force that is transferred from the concrete back to your body. When walking on level ground, you're exerting about 1.5 times your body weight on your joints. So you're exerting 300 pounds of force on every joint. When you run, that force can be as much as five times your weight. So that same person is exerting half a ton of force on their ankles, knees, and hips.

It's quite incredible, really. The human body can endure a lot of abuse. But as you can imagine, the heavier you are, the faster that cartilage will deteriorate. And to reference Wolff's Law mentioned earlier, when there are extreme forces exerted on the body, the body will react to it. In this case, the body will produce new bone. This is how arthritis becomes debilitating, and the joint will ultimately need to be replaced.

My advice to those facing arthritic joints: Maintain a normal weight and develop a game plan with your orthopedist. Try every intervention possible, e.g., joint injections, platelet rich plasma (PRP), exosomes, peptides, stem cells, everything you can get your hands on before getting a joint replacement. I don't have anything against those procedures; I've helped with plenty of them and see many success stories. But you want to delay that surgery for as long as possible.

I hope this chapter has provided you with some practical knowledge and know-how when it comes to bones and joints. The upside to these injuries is that overwhelmingly, there's a solution for the problem. I encourage you to do your research on surgeons and therapists long before you ever need them. Write their names and contact info on your EAP. I hope you never need them.

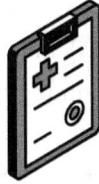

# CHAPTER 11

## KIDS AREN'T JUST LITTLE ADULTS

*A man's health can be judged by which he takes two at a time–pills or stairs.*

–Joan Welsh

As I've gotten older, I've become more of a medical consultant at motocross races as opposed to the young cowboy running all over the track, picking riders up as they ultimately taste test the various terrain. In case you didn't know, I've provided medical coverage for the American Motorcyclist Association (AMA) and AMA Pro Racing since 2005. I would travel all over the country and stand on the side of a professional motorcycle track, waiting for someone to fall off and get hurt. Unfortunately, that happens more often than not in this field. I definitely stayed busy on weekends at the track.

One day I was helping a good friend of mine with a big race at his track near my home. He told me that he "had the medical covered" but requested I carry a radio "just in case." He had a fleet of EMTs (Emergency Medical Technicians) and medical personnel on location, and he did a spectacular job at planning for emergencies in order to keep his riders safe.

He could not have planned for what happened to this little boy on this day.

The child could not have been nine years old, but you'd never know by how he was riding (more like piloting) his bike. This kid was literally flying. As I was walking around the track, I noticed a bit of commotion at the top of a hill, followed by a lot of anxious chatter on the radio.

"Arden!" I heard over the headset. "We need you over here!" I picked up my pace.

As I'm speeding on this four-wheeler over to the crowd, I'm counting all the EMTs that are already on the scene. I usually just stay out of their way as a general courtesy. I wouldn't expect them to barge into a treatment room at my office, so I like to show them the same respect. But as I was getting the story, I couldn't help but intervene.

This young hotshot was in the middle of the track, in a landing zone of a blind jump, and the technician was about to cut his pants off on the track.

I'm thinking, this is super serious, we need to red flag the race, we need to call a helicopter... all the bad things start pouring into my head.

I get to the screaming child.

"Don't cut my pants!" he screams. He's anxious and panting, but he doesn't seem to be in a lot of pain.

I push past the seemingly fresh-out-of-school technician. "Where are you hurt, dude? Where is your pain?" I asked, yelling over the noise of the machines and crowd of people.

The child grabs his leg and gives it a shake. "Right here!" As he jiggles his tiny thigh, he's still yelling and anxious.

I performed a quick assessment and told him, "Tell ya what; if you can stand up and walk off the track, I won't cut your pants off."

Immediately, he stopped with the tears, hopped up, grabbed his helmet, and trotted off the track with only the slightest hobble.

"How'd you do that?" The EMT asked me with a perplexed look on his face. "I thought he broke his leg by all the screaming!"

"How many kids do you have?" I asked.

"Well, none. I haven't dealt with a ton of kids at work either."

"Gotta love 'em!" I chuckled as I patted him on the shoulder.

I wanted to start with this story to relay the point that *things aren't always what they seem.* There's a saying in medicine that "kids aren't small adults," meaning, you can't just treat a kid like a three-foot tall adult. Talking louder to them as if they can't hear will probably not get you very far. I'm writing this chapter to offer you my experience getting kids on your side, keeping them safe and *not* becoming deathly afraid of the medical profession.

There are certainly instances where kids and kid illnesses can be scary. But with "common things being common," children are, by design, a very resilient human form. Thinking about it from an evolutionary perspective, children *must* be resilient, or the human species would have never flourished.

This is often forgotten. Combine that with typical American medical practices determined to treat everything, and you have a society that medicates kids who probably don't need more than a hug and some sleep.

I understand there's a spectrum to everything. That is what brings me to my first point about kids: If kids are sick, usually they will be "unsick" in a matter of a few days, no matter what you do about it.

As a parent, it's okay to take a deep breath and know that, if we're looking at the odds, this will blow over in a few days without too much of a fuss. So instead of having to make overnight phone calls for little Johnny's 100.1 F fever, it's okay to give him a cool rag for his forehead, or perhaps some liquid ibuprofen, if appropriate. And then you monitor him. Time will tell you a lot when it comes to kids.

Another thing I've learned—both as a clinician and a parent—is that really sick kids don't fake it. I currently have a six-year old child who recently learned that "being sick" can keep you home instead of going to school. So about once a week, he'll come downstairs and complain of his head or tummy hurting. It's always something you can't *really* look at; adults do this too.

I typically tell him that he picked the wrong parents on which to try to pull medical stunts but one day, as his older brother was getting ready for school, he wasn't coming down the stairs in his usual hurricane fashion. He wasn't coming down the stairs at all.

So, I go up to his room to get him ready, and all I see in bed is this sick child. You can probably close your eyes and visualize a kid that looked like mine that morning, i.e., pale, clammy, eyes barely open, curled up in a ball, shivering yet sweating. That was my kid. The first thing I did (whether I knew it or not) was determine whether he was *really* sick or *faking* sick. This kid was definitely sick.

That's an important step, and something you should do every time you assess a kid. Because this step is fundamental to what you do next, and your answer can change over time.

The next step is to determine how sick the child is. Remember, usually it's going to be a "wait and see" situation. Most children at this age suffer from viral illnesses that self-limit. When you bring kids with viruses to the local urgent care or their pediatrician's office, they will give you a number of helpful items or suggestions like a list of OTC medications, supplements, or remedies, and they will tell you when to return or go to the local ER. They usually won't just determine what the child is experiencing, nor will they offer anything that you cannot obtain on your own, such as a prescription medication.

I stand corrected. *Some* pediatricians and urgent care providers will dump antibiotics in your lap. I've already given my opinion on these "practitioners" and will only say again that if this is your experience, then you should probably find a new provider.

Knowing this, I want to know *exactly* what this child is experiencing, such as what's hurting, when does it hurt, how long has it hurt, does it hurt all the time or just sometimes, is there anything else going on, etc.

If the symptoms sound like a cold, then it's probably a cold. If you recall Chapter 8: Bacteria vs. Virus (vs. Allergies), overwhelmingly, we don't have a lot of "fix it now" treatments for viruses, especially for the common cold. Obviously, we can all identify five or 10 "cold beaters" that we've seen on commercials or browsed past in our local pharmacy or grocery store. But let me assure you: If that little box or bottle really cured a common cold, it'd be in every medicine cabinet on Earth.

Big pharma knows this. Recently, there was a class action suit filed[39] against the big pharma manufacturers in late 2023 because they all falsely claimed the drug phenylephrine–a popular decongestant ingredient– would solve all your problems related to the common cold. The kicker is that these companies knew that the ingredient was no better than a placebo, based on data from various studies.

That doesn't mean we are helpless in making our little ones feel better. We just have to understand what our objective is when giving children, or adults for that matter, any type of supplement or medication.

Symptom control. That's the main goal when my kids come to me with cold and flu symptoms. Control the symptoms, keep the kid comfortable, and avoid secondary illnesses.

So, if you go to the pharmacy, and you're looking for kids' medication, I ask you make a couple of commonsense decisions. First, make sure you have a way to properly weigh the child. If you don't have a scale at home, see if there's one at your pharmacy. One is usually somewhere in there, especially if they do pharmacy consults. An accurate weight will determine the proper dose of medication for your child. We don't want to guess. Too little, and you're wasting time and money, and your kid doesn't feel any better. Too much, and your kid can possibly overdose.

Second, if it's a liquid, use a syringe. If one is not provided, ask the pharmacy for one. They'll be happy to give one to you. This goes back to guessing. I've never met a parent who can accurately describe exactly how much medication is in one of those little cups that come with liquid medication.

As far as what medications to give to kids. This is a loaded topic that will inevitably get me some hostile responses. Who would have thought that medication selection would be a polarizing topic, but alas, here we are.

I don't give my kids, nor do I recommend to my patients, Tylenol® or any form of acetaminophen. There's enough suspicion surrounding this drug to make people scratch their heads and question its safety. If you don't know, just Google "acetaminophen lawsuit" or "acetaminophen red 40."

I also don't give my kids a bunch of NSAIDS like Motrin®. If you remember me talking about the inflammatory process, we need some inflammation to help us heal. So, the more appropriate thing to do is to modulate the inflammation. Truthfully, that might be easier to do with an ankle sprain than a head cold, so I do use it. But I try to use it sparingly. I seek noninvasive alternatives, depending on the symptoms I'm treating.

Aspirin has been linked to Reye's Syndrome in kids, so that's an absolute no-no.

For congestion, I don't think there's anything better than diluting that congestion with saline. Water is the best expectorant known to man, and there's not a drug in any pharmacy that can come close. I recommend products like NeilMed® Sinus Rinse [40, 41,42, 43] to irrigate nasal congestion. This will also help unclog ears and potentially decrease the risk for secondary bacterial ear infections. There are other suction products[44] out there also that'll suck and irrigate at the same time.

I've mentioned the word "secondary" a couple of times now. Remember me saying there's not much to do about viruses? Well, that's still true, but one of the issues on our list of goals is to prevent an environment ripe for bacterial growth. This is how viruses can morph into bacterial infections.

Take little Johnny's earache, for example. Overwhelmingly, this begins as congestion from allergies or a viral illness of some kind. The inflammatory process commences, and a flood of mucus gets trapped behind the tympanic membrane, i.e., your eardrum. As that mucus sits and pools, it's creating an inviting environment, that is dark, warm, and moist, perfect for bacteria to flourish. Before you know it, there's pus, pain, hearing loss, and more swelling. A virus evolved into a bacterial infection.

Even still, in cases like this, the literature is trending more towards a "watch and wait" approach to ear infections in kids. Not all ear infections require treatment with antibiotics. As I'm writing this chapter, I've been treating one of my kid's ear infections conservatively, without prescription medication, while another one needed antibiotics.

As the parent, the layperson, use time as your guide. Do all you can to prevent it, via irrigation, chest rubs, homeopathy, etc., and give it two- to three days. If pain persists or worsens, then you have your answer as to how to proceed.

In the following paragraphs, I'm going to bold type the topic for your reference. I'm going to rapid fire some suggestions that have been given to me by my colleagues in pediatrics from across the country.

**Pediatric sleep apnea** is a real thing, and it's not "cute." Chronic snoring kids should be assessed for airway issues, infected/hypertrophied tonsils, or other airway issues. If they're sick/congested and snoring, no need to rush to the ER. We know the temporary cause. But if you notice the issue occurring more frequently, particularly when they're not sick, then get them checked out. Other signs include the child complaining of being tired all the time, crankiness, more frequently falling asleep during the day, etc.

Batteries—especially the shiny button batteries—are very attractive to infants and toddlers. Let me tell you; it's not fun having to retrieve that from a kid's GI tract. It's a medical emergency that in large part, should be avoided by properly securing the home beforehand. I'd rather a kid swallow a marble or a quarter any day over a battery.

This leads me to **childproofing your home.** If you're a parent with a curious, walking toddler, make a little checklist. Don't reinvent the wheel; Google search for one, and you'll get 42 million choices. Common items to childproof include outlets, blinds (cordless are preferred), medications, weapons (including kitchen knives in lower drawers), treadmills or other workout equipment, chemicals and cleaning supplies, pet food, and bathrooms. Develop small habits that include keeping bedroom and bathroom doors closed, and invest in locks for kitchen and bathroom cabinets. I like those magnetic kits that adhere to the inside of the cabinet doors.[45]

**Kids can drown in next to no water.** Kids under four require special attention here. Pools obviously need to be secured, and most homeowner's insurance policies now require some sort of child protection, like a perimeter fence. Kids can drown in toilets, buckets, and sinks, so as I mentioned, keep them off limits. I recommend swimming lessons at an age earlier than you would normally think. In other words, if they can walk, they can take swimming lessons.

**Infants don't need water or cow's milk.** Stick to formula or breast milk until at least six months for water (even then, a small amount), and 12 months for cow's milk (there's no rush there).

**Don't share a bed with your baby.** I wish this one was more obvious, but bad accidents can happen. Babies can fall asleep on your chest; it's one of the best feelings on Earth. But before you go to bed, put them in their own sleeping area for their safety.

**Car seats.**[46] Entire books have been written on this subject alone. There are certain parameters for car seats, and it goes by the age, height, and weight of the child. It's imperative that your child is fitted in the appropriate car seat. The hospital won't let you leave without one, and it's just the safe thing to do. Read the manual when you get it. You'd be surprised that those instructions tell you all you need to know about your new device. If you're still confused, most police stations and fire departments will help you install it correctly.

**Helmets** are an obvious accessory to many sports and recreational activities. Not all helmets are created equally. As a medical professional who advocates for motorcycle riding and racing, I want to outfit my riders in the most appropriate gear and equipment possible, and that includes proper fit. Fit is more important than the quality of the helmet, in my opinion. Helmets should be snug but not painful. They should not move up and down, side to side when appropriately fitted. Remember that most helmet companies will sell different pads to insert inside the shell to ensure the best fit. This will reduce the risk of concussion or severe injury in the event of an accident.

It should go without saying that if you're on a bike or motorized vehicle, put a helmet on. In all my career, I haven't seen a battle between skull and pavement, tree branch or other hard surface where the skull actually won. Protect your head.

**If you have guns in your home**, go over the universal firearm rules. Depending on their age, you could introduce them to Eddie Eagle, The National Rifle Association's cartoon spokesperson to inform kids and parents about gun safety.[47] There's a great video on their website instructing kids what to do:

- STOP!
- Don't touch
- Run away
- Tell an adult

I'm also a fan of not keeping weapons and firearms a big secret in the home. If you're a gun owner, it's necessary that you're well-versed in all the gun safety terms and protocols, so show your kids the weapon and tell them about it. If they're curious, ensure the weapon is unloaded, and present it to them. Let them handle it, and teach them about it. Take the mystery away so they don't go looking for it when you're not home.

**Talk to your kids about vaping, smoking, drinking, and drug use.** Similar to the gun talk, take the mystery away and they'll be less likely to try these substances behind your back. That doesn't mean you let them try them. But by introducing the topic in a conversation, there's less illusion and mystery. I tell my kids why I don't smoke, vape, or do drugs. If I have a drink, which is seldom, I frequently will have age-appropriate discussions with them about it.

The consequences are dire. I've seen kids really mess themselves up with "harmless" vaping, and drug use is an entirely different tragedy that we'd all like to avoid with our children. Keep the dialogue open, and create an environment that's welcoming and open to all sorts of questions.

Remember that kids aren't little adults. They have developing brains and aren't capable of complex thought or action. Also remember that humans as a species would not have made it this far without having resilient offspring. Thankfully, most childhood illnesses will self-limit. Deep breath, mom or dad. You can do this; your child's life could depend on it.

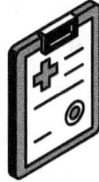

# CHAPTER 12

## THE END OF THE BEGINNING

*Disease is the biggest money maker in our economy.*

–John H. Tobe

I didn't fully believe that quote until I started working in the healthcare industry. There are a significant number of well-intentioned people with hearts of gold that work in the medical community. Some of the most selfless, thoughtful, caring people I've ever met wear white coats and stethoscopes around their neck. Most of the people who decide on medicine as a career fit that description. They want to help people. The problem is that the industry gets in the way of legitimate "care."

People are paying for insurance plans only to be told that the drug they need isn't covered under their plan. Providers are telling loved ones of patients "there's nothing they can do" when all opportunities haven't been considered, or alternatives are viewed as "extreme." Hospital administrators are more concerned about room turnover than the care of the lives lying in that room. The business of medicine destroys otherwise good-meaning people trying to make a difference.

It's more important now more than ever that you educate yourself and be mindful of what's going on around you. It starts with self-care, and it continues with knowing how the game is played. The industry intentionally makes the rules of the game complicated so that you don't feel like you're even playing. But when *you* understand what's going on, you can be a threat to their profit. Even more important, you can be an advocate for yourself and your loved ones to ensure you get the care you expect.

I recently lost someone in my family that received "questionable" care at a facility. Prior to their passing, this person's daughter called me in a panic and explained the current situation. The patient was in remission from cancer and was doing well. One day, they awoke with progressive numbness in their extremities and eventually became nonresponsive. The patient was brought to her doctor's ER and was quickly brought back for evaluation. The daughter told me that she never saw the treating physician, only a resident, who told her to start preparing the patient's "final wishes," and that there was simply nothing they could do.

Prior to this situation, the patient was not scanned, no labs were drawn, no differential diagnosis was presented. There was no communication with the family.

On my call with the patient's daughter, I suggested that she transfer her mother to another facility in the area, one known to have an excellent neurology department.

Upon her request, she was flooded with a team of physicians, surgeons, and hospital staff. Now they wanted to talk. Now they were offering all sorts of treatment plans and suggestions, and they were much more willing to offer assistance to her mom. I stressed that they should still get her transferred, as time was precious.

She was eventually transferred, and within an hour of the transfer, it was noted on a CT scan that the patient had severe swelling on her brain.

An emergency craniotomy was performed, and the next morning, the patient was able to sit up, hug her daughter, and have a brief conversation.

I was in tears the next day when I heard this news over the phone. This brief moment proved to be her last moment with her daughter, as the reduction in swelling was only temporary. The swelling continued, eventually leading to her passing.

Can you comprehend what that morning meant to this patient's daughter? Do you know how many people do not get that opportunity? Why couldn't the first hospital offer a similar treatment option, and would the time saved turned into a different outcome for the patient?

Regardless of the details of the case, this is an example of why I wrote this book. If I can empower one person to change one outcome, this was worth it.

Let me emphasize that the medical community is not some big, bad machine out to get you. I do believe that we are witnessing some nefarious acts in sectors of the medical community, but I do believe that most people are trying to do good by their fellow man and go home with a paycheck to feed their families.

This does *not* change the fact that it's a system designed to make money. And you must be prepared for this fact. Whether it's you, your child, your parent, a loved one, or a dear friend in that hospital bed, someone needs to understand with the rules of the game. You need to play ball, and I suggest you lace up, take a deep breath and get ready to play hard.

I firmly believe there are many ways to tell people a message you're trying to convey, and you certainly get a more positive response with honey rather than vinegar. That said, I had no problems recommending to my friend's daughter that she tell the hospital staff to kindly transfer the patient, or her attorney will demand the transfer.

After completing this book (and doing a little research on your own), you'll now be equipped with your personal "Homemade MD." You can hang this on your wall as your diploma if you choose, but this book gives you zero chance of becoming a doctor. It wasn't intended to do so. I hope you take away from this book a sense of understanding. A sense of confidence. Know that there are people on your side willing to help you make a difference in your own life.

The best thing you can do now is continue to learn and be the provider that your loved ones need you to be. Prepare your EAP, stock your medicine cabinet, and question everything you read in medical literature. If you have suggestions for future books, I'm all ears. Please send me your feedback and topics you'd like to know more about.

It's critical to be a healthcare advocate for yourself and your loved ones. The knowledge you have and the questions you ask could be the difference between a life saved and a life lost.

# ACKNOWLEDGMENTS

To my amazing family: Katherine, Kayden, Karsen, and Klaire. You bring me inspiration every day to be a better human. I love you with every cell in my body. Thank you for putting up with my often manic thought processes. You're all more than I could ever deserve.

To Greg Anderson and Greg Lapin. Whether you knew it or not, you guys inspired me to put my thoughts to paper, and more importantly, to see it through. Thank you for showing me the importance of doing hard things, and thank you for reminding me that "no one is coming to save you."

Thanks to my colleagues, the providers who trained me and the staff that helped me help others. Many of you helped me write this book in between patients and after hours. I'm so thankful to have worked with some of the best humans medicine has to offer.

To my patients... Thank you for putting your trust in me. To those that took my advice and made one change in their life, their actions are why I chose to be a provider. I now understand that there are those who simply choose not to help themselves; I just pray that, one day, you'll remember some silly analogy I told you and change your ways.

# ABOUT THE AUTHOR

Arden Ballard, MS, PA-C, ATC is a child of God, a husband, a father, a business owner, and a practicing physician assistant in Mandeville, Louisiana. He never had a desire to write a book until he was completely burnt out in his position treating urgent care patients. He always wanted to help people, but ironically, he felt that the system he joined to help people only seemed to get in his way of doing so.

Now, alongside his lovely wife, Katherine, Arden owns his own medical practice and helps regular people be their own healthcare advocate. Whether it's a mom trying to do the best for their child, or an adult caring for their elderly parents, everyone needs a guide in this ever-changing and complex medical system we have in the U.S.

When Arden isn't working, he's playing with his children: Kayden, Karsen, and Klaire, and his two dogs, Sadie and Marly.

# URGENT PLEA!

**Thank You For Reading My Book!**
I really appreciate all of your feedback and
I love hearing what you have to say.

I need your input to make the next version of this
book and my future books better.

Please take two minutes now to leave a helpful review on
Amazon letting me know what you thought of the book:

thehomemademd.com/review
Thanks so much!
–Arden

# BIBLIOGRAPHY

1. Darabon, Frank (director), 1999, "The Green Mile," Warner Hollywood Studios.

2. Sweeney, J.F. (2019). Physician retirement: Why it's hard for doctors to retire. Medical Economics. https://www.medicaleconomics. com/view/physician-retirement-why-its-hard-doctors-retire

3. Healthline. https://www.healthline.com/health-news/policy-ten-administrators-for-every-one-us-doctor-092813 (article no longer available).

4. Case Management Society of America (CMSA). What is a case manager? https://cmsa.org/who-we-are/what-is-a-case-manager/

5. Davis. E. (2023). Duties and types of case managers. verywellhealth. https://www.verywellhealth.com/what-does-a-case-manager-do-1738560#toc-health-insurance-case-manager

6. USC Suzanne Dworak-Peck School of Social Work. (2018). What do medical social workers do? https://dworakpeck.usc.edu/news/what-do-medical-social-workers-do

7. Columbia University. Allopathic Medicine - Overview of the Profession. https://www.ccseas.columbia.edu/preprofessional/health/types/allopathic.php#:~:text=Allopathic%20medicine%20refers%20to%20a,orthodox%20medicine%2C%20and%20Western%20medicine

8. NENA The 9-1-1 Association. 9-1-1 Origin & History. https://www.nena.org/page/911overviewfacts

9. NENA The 9-1-1 Association. 9-1-1 Statistics. https://www.nena.org/page/911Statistics#:~:text=9%2D1%2D1%20Call%20Volume,in%20the%20U.S.%20each%20year

10. Los Angeles Almanac. Using 911 in Los Angeles County. http://www.laalmanac.com/communications/cm01x.php

11. Los Angeles Almanac. Using 911 in Los Angeles County. http://www.laalmanac.com/communications/cm01x.php

12. Walden University. 10 Things You Might Not Know About the United States' 911 Emergency Telephone Number. https://www.waldenu.edu/online-masters-programs/ms-in-criminal-justice/resource/ten-things-you-might-not-know-about-the-united-states-911-emergency-telephone-number#:~:text=In%20an%20average%20year%2C%20around,However%20%E2%80%A6&text=People%20call%20911%20for%20all,Overflowing%20toilets

13. Davis, M. (2023). Ambulance spending for medicare beneficiaries totaled $3.95 billion in 2021 — Down 3.9% from 2020 and the lowest in 10 Years.

https://www.valuepenguin.com/cost-ambulance-services#:~:text=Than%20%2446%20Billion-,Ambulance%20Rides%20Have%20Cost%20%241%2C189%20on%20Average%20Since,Totaling%20More%20Than%20%2446%20Billion&text=Ambulance%2Drelated%20spending%20for%20Medicare,annually%20from%202010%20to%202019.&text=The%20cost%20of%20an%20ambulance,average%20of%20%241%2C189%20a%20year.

14. Brayne, A.B., Brayne, R.P., Fowler, A.J. (2021) Medical specialties and life expectancy: An analysis of doctors' obituaries 1997–2019. Lifestyle Medicine.

https://onlinelibrary.wiley.com/doi/full/10.1002/lim2.23#:~:text=The%20specialties%20with%20the%20youngest,did%20not%20differ%20by%20specialty

15. Mental Health Resource Center.

https://www.webmd.com/mental-health/news/20180508/doctors-suicide-rate-highest-of-any-profession

16. CompleteCare. (2018). The History of Urgent Care. https://www.visitcompletecare.com/blog/history-of-urgent-care/

17. Statista. Number of urgent care centers in the U.S. from 2013 to 2019. https://www.statista.com/statistics/908860/number-of-us-urgent-care-centers/

18. https://symptomate.com/

19. Tardi, C. (2021). Healthcare Power of Attorney (HCPA): Definition and how to set up. Investopedia. Healthcare Power of Attorney (HCPA): Definition and How To Set Up.
    https://www.investopedia.com/terms/h/hcpa.asp

20. Smith, L. (2023). What Is a Will, What Does It Cover, and Why Do I Need One? Investopedia.
    https://www.investopedia.com/articles/pf/08/what-is-a-will.asp

21. IBIS World. (2023). Pharmacies & Drug Stores in the US - Market Size (2004–2029)
    https://www.ibisworld.com/industry-statistics/market-size/pharmacies-drug-stores-united-states/#:~:text=The%20market%20size%2C%20measured%20by,is%20%24346.3bn%20in%202022

22. Statista.Top U.S. pharmacies ranked by prescription drugs market share in 2022.
    https://www.statista.com/statistics/734171/pharmacies-ranked-by-rx-market-share-in-us/

23. Seeley, E., Singh, S. (2021). Competition, consolidation, and evolution in the pharmacy market. The Commonwealth Fund.
    https://www.commonwealthfund.org/publications/issue-briefs/2021/aug/competition-consolidation-evolution-pharmacy-market

24. (2023) Pharmacy benefit managers. NAIC.
    https://content.naic.org/cipr_topics/topic_pharmacy_benefit_managers.htm

25. https://drinklmnt.com/

26. Suzuki, M., Yamada, K., Nagao, M., Aoki, E., Matsumoto, M., Hirayama, T., et al. (2011). Antimicrobial ointments and methicillin resistant Staphylococcus aureus USA300.
https://wwwnc.cdc.gov/eid/pdfs/10-1365-ahead_of_print.pdf

27. John Y Chung, J.Y., Herbert, M.E. (2021). Myth: silver sulfadiazine is the best treatment for minor burns. Western Journal of Medicine.
https://www.ncbi.nlm.nih.gov/pmc/articles/PMC1071544/

28. Jase Medical. Medical Preparedness.
https://jasemedical.com/

29. Gomstyn, A. What's an HSA, and why should you have one? Aetna.
https://www.aetna.com/health-guide/can-pay-hsa.html

30. Whitwam, R. (2013). Simulating 1 second of human brain activity takes 82,944 processors. ET.
https://www.extremetech.com/extreme/163051-simulating-1-second-of-human-brain-activity-takes-82944-processors

31. The history of antibiotics. Microbiology Society.
https://microbiologysociety.org/members-outreach-resources/outreach-resources/antibiotics-unearthed/antibiotics-and-antibiotic-resistance/the-history-of-antibiotics.html

32. Gelman, L. (2022). 10 wildly overinflated hospital costs you didn't know about. The Healthy.
https://www.thehealthy.com/healthcare/health-insurance/wildly-overinflated-hospital-costs

33. Wyckoff, A.S. (ed). (2016). FDA proposes limit on arsenic in infant rice cereals. American Academy of Pediatrics
https://publications.aap.org/aapnews/news/9164?autologincheck=redirected?nfToken=00000000-0000-0000-0000-000000000000

34. (2022). Highly processed foods can share the addictive qualities of tobacco, researchers say. Virginia Tech.
https://news.vt.edu/articles/2022/11/HPFsandtobacco_fralinbiomed_1109.html

35. (2022). 11 foods that boost your immune system. Cleveland Clinic.
https://health.clevelandclinic.org/food-to-boost-your-immune-system/

36. Asher, G.N., Corbett, A.H., Hawke, R.L. (2017). Common herbal dietary supplement–Drug interactions. American Family Physician.
https://www.aafp.org/pubs/afp/issues/2017/0715/p101.html

37. Elnaggar, S. What to know about tissue healing timelines. PREHAB.
https://theprehabguys.com/tissue-healing-timelines/#

38. How long will this take? Time frames of tissue healing. Cambridge Osteopathy (pub).
https://cambridgeosteopathy.co.uk/2018/11/01/how-long-will-this-take-time-frames-of-tissue-healing/

39. Stempel, J. J&J unit, P&G, Walgreens misled consumers about decongestants, lawsuits say

https://www.reuters.com/legal/jj-pg-sued-after-fda-panel-ruling-cold-medicine-decongestant-2023-09-14/

40. https://amzn.to/40FkzG2

41. https://amzn.to/3R1Nvoo

42. https://amzn.to/47hzkBf

43. https://amzn.to/40FPMc0

44. https://amzn.to/40FPMc0

45. https://amzn.to/47GFZEC

46. Car Seats: Information for Families. American Academy of Pediatrics.

https://www.healthychildren.org/English/safety-prevention/on-the-go/Pages/Car-Safety-Seats-Information-for-Families.aspx

47. Talking to your child about gun safety. NRA Explore.
https://eddieeagle.nra.org/pa

www.ingramcontent.com/pod-product-compliance
Lightning Source LLC
Chambersburg PA
CBHW062100270326
41931CB00013B/3158